NCLEX-RN

Practice Test and Review

The Chicago Review Press

NCLEX-RN

Practice Test and Review

Linda Waide, MSN, MEd, RN and
Berta Roland, MSN, RN

CHICAGO REVIEW PRESS

Library of Congress Cataloging-in Publication Data

Waide, Linda.
    The Chicago Review Press NCLEX-RN practice test and review / Linda Waide and Berta Roland.
    p.   cm.
    ISBN 1-55652-328-9 (alk. paper)
    1. Nursing—Examinations, questions, etc.   I. Roland, Berta. II. Title.
RT52.W34   1998
610.73'076'93076—DC21

                                        98-29573

                                                            CIP

Published by Chicago Review Press, Incorporated
814 North Franklin Street
Chicago, Illinois 60610

ISBN 1-55652-328-9
Printed in the United States of America
5 4 3 2 1

Contents

Introduction

A General Description of the NCLEX-RN

This book is designed to provide you, a candidate for registered nurse licensure, with as much information as possible about the examination that is part of the process of licensing nurses in the United States.

The examination is the National Council Licensure Examination for Registered Nurses, more commonly known as the NCLEX-RN. It is a requirement for initial licensure in each of the United States, the District of Columbia, and the U.S. territories of Guam, the Virgin Islands, American Samoa, and the Commonwealth of Northern Mariana Islands.

The National Council of State Boards of Nursing, Inc.

The organization responsible for preparing the NCLEX-RN and its counterpart for licensed practical nurses, the NCLEX-PN, is the National Council of State Boards of Nursing, Inc. NCLEX, NCLEX-RN, and NCLEX-PN are registered trademarks of the National Council of State Boards of Nursing, Inc. Founded in 1978, the National Council consists of 62 member boards of nursing, all of whom have been given responsibility by their state legislatures to regulate nursing practice in their own states. That responsibility includes not only regulating the practice of nurses already licensed but also determining who may enter into the practice of nursing.

Entry into the practice of nursing, as with any licensed profession, is regulated by each state for the purpose of protecting the public from those who are unable to practice nursing safely and effectively. Therefore, candidates for licensure are asked by boards of nursing to provide evidence of their ability to deliver effective nursing care.

The NCLEX-RN

The primary evidence requires, along with a degree or diploma from a board-approved nursing education program, the successful completion of the NCLEX-RN, which has been developed by the National Council under the direction of its member boards to test a licensure candidate's capabilities for safe and effective nursing practice at the entry level. It is designed to test essential nursing knowledge by asking you to apply that knowledge to health-care situations demanding nursing intervention.

You are already probably well prepared for such an examination. You have completed a course of instruction for students whose goal is to become registered nurses. You have learned the basic information necessary to practice safe and effective nursing through various kinds of classroom activities and clinical practice, along with your own study, as determined by each nursing education program's faculty. And you have taken examinations constructed to determine whether or not you have acquired the necessary knowledge and developed an understanding of clinical practice.

That educational process is an excellent preparation for the NCLEX-RN. The NCLEX examinations are written by faculty members from nursing education programs around the country, along with clinical practitioners from a full range of practice areas and settings who supervise recently graduated nurses. Some of your own teachers and clinical supervisors may have been asked, at one time or another, to serve in a writing session for the NCLEX-RN.

The NCLEX-RN Using CAT

In April 1994, the NCLEX-RN changed from a full-day, pencil-and-paper examination that was offered twice a year to a computerized examination lasting 5 hours or less that can be taken year-round at the candidate's convenience. The NCLEX-RN using CAT, or Computerized Adaptive Testing, is administered by the Educational Testing Service (ETS) at Sylvan Technology Centers. These are small, modern facilities with up to 15 testing stations each, located for the most part in shopping areas with ample parking and nearby public transportation. Every state and territory has at least one testing center, and many, of course, have more.

The NCLEX-RN is offered by appointment up to 15 hours a day at most centers, 6 days per week, and on Sundays when necessary to meet peak demand. Examination results are sent electronically to your board of nursing within 48 hours of the examination. Each board maintains its own schedule for releasing results to candidates. Testing centers do not release examination results, and results are not available by phone. As in the past, failing candidates will receive a diagnostic profile with their results to help them pinpoint areas of weakness.

How Do I Schedule the NCLEX-RN?

Candidates apply directly to their board of nursing for authorization to take the NCLEX-RN. For your convenience, a list of all the boards of nursing with their addresses and phone numbers is provided at the end of this introduction. The board of nursing will send you a candidate bulletin containing a registration form and information about the examination. When your application has been approved and your registration processed, you will receive an Authorization to Test form and scheduling information from ETS. At that time, you may phone the Sylvan Technology Center where you want to take the examination to schedule an appointment. Eligible first-time candidates will be offered an appointment within 30 days; eligible repeat candidates within 45 days.

The Basics of the NCLEX-RN Using CAT

The NCLEX-RN using CAT consists of multiple-choice questions with 4 possible answers. The entire question and its answer choices fit completely on the computer screen (see diagram). Only two keys are used to take the examination—the space bar and the enter key. All the other keys on the computer keyboard are deactivated, or turned off, during the examination. The space bar moves the cursor among the answer choices. To record an answer and bring up the next question, you strike the enter key twice.

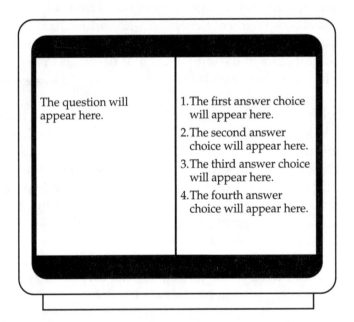

Candidates sometimes fear that they will not do well on the NCLEX-RN if they do not have computer experience. Research has shown that this is not true. All candidates take a keyboard tutorial with a practice exercise before the examination begins, and attendants are available to answer questions about the computer throughout the examination.

What Are the Advantages of CAT?

For you, the NCLEX-RN using CAT offers the possibility of year-round licensure as well as a shorter, more convenient test. For both you and the licensing authorities, it provides a more efficient measurement of nursing competence than was possible with the paper-and-pencil examination. The computer begins the test with an easy question. If you answer correctly, a more difficult question appears on the screen. If you answer incorrectly, an easier question is offered next. Questions are offered until you have been tested in each area required by the overall test plan and have answered enough questions that a pass or fail decision can be made, until you run out of time, or until you have taken the maximum number of questions—205 on the NCLEX-RN. No passing candidate will answer fewer than 85 questions, and no candidate will answer more than 205 questions over 5 hours of testing.

Is CAT Fair?

Yes. Computerized adaptive testing automatically adjusts to the competence level of each candidate. Candidates who are far above or far below the passing standard for the NCLEX-RN will answer fewer questions. Those whose competence is closer to the passing standard will answer more questions. The NCLEX-RN stops when the 5-hour time limit is reached, when the maximum number of questions have been answered, or when enough questions have been answered that a pass or fail decision can be made with at least 95% confidence. It is to your advantage to pace yourself during the examination as if you will have to take the maximum number of items. Remember, though, that some passing candidates will answer more questions and some will answer fewer questions. The same will be true for failing candidates. All candidates will have ample opportunity to demonstrate their competence to practice nursing at the entry level.

How Is the Pass-Fail Decision Made?

You will pass the NCLEX-RN if you satisfy 1 of the following 3 conditions:
1. You answer at least the minimum number of questions within the time allowed and your competence measure is significantly above the passing standard.
2. You answer the maximum number of questions within the time allowed and your competence measure is above the passing standard.
3. You answer test questions for the maximum time allowed, you answer at least the minimum number of questions, and your competence measure is above the passing standard for all of the last 60 questions.

You will fail the examination if:
1. You answer at least the minimum number of questions in the time allowed and your competence measure is significantly below the passing standard.
2. You answer the maximum number of questions in the time allowed and your competence measure is below the passing standard.
3. You answer questions for the maximum time allowed, you answer at least the minimum number of questions, and your competence measure falls below the passing standard for any of the last 60 questions.
4. You have not answered the minimum number of questions in the maximum time of 5 hours.

It may reassure you to know that 85 to 93% of first-time, U.S.-educated candidates pass the NCLEX-RN.

Can I Skip, Review, or Change My Answers in the NCLEX-RN?

No. Because the way you answer one question to a large extent determines what your next question will be, there is no point in being able to return to an earlier question. If you answer a question incorrectly, the next question that appears on the screen is less difficult, and your chance of answering correctly increases. The CAT method protects you from "digging yourself into a hole" of wrong answers from which you cannot escape. Don't worry if you change your mind about an answer after you have recorded it on the examination.

Are Breaks Allowed During the NCLEX-RN?

After 2 hours of testing, everyone takes a mandatory 10-minute break. After an additional hour and a half of testing, you may take a second scheduled break if you wish. Candidates can take unscheduled breaks at any time. All breaks and the brief keyboard tutorial are included in the 5-hour time limit.

Review and Challenge of the NCLEX-RN

In certain states and territories, failing candidates are permitted by law to review their examinations and challenge their results. Such reviews are conducted at a Sylvan Technology Center; a fee is charged. For more information, contact your board of nursing.

The Test Questions

All of the questions on the NCLEX-RN are multiple-choice with 4 answers to choose from. The initial part of a multiple-choice question is called the *stem*, and it is the stem that states the question being asked. Three of the choices, which are not correct, are called *distractors*. Each distractor will seem plausible until the student thinks critically about it. For example, read the sample question below.

0 - 0

A 4-month-old is to be weighed daily. At which of the following times would it be best for the nurse to weigh the infant?

1. prior to the first morning feeding
2. after the infant has been bathed
3. after the infant's first bowel movement of the day
4. whenever the mother is available to assist with the procedure

In this question, the background is "A four-month-old is to be weighed daily." The question is "At which of the following times would it be best for the nurse to weigh the infant?" and the correct answer is "prior to the first morning feeding." The other answers are distractors.

The Chicago Review Press NCLEX-RN Practice Test and Review

The Chicago Review Press NCLEX-RN Practice Test and Review was developed specifically for nursing students preparing for the NCLEX-RN. It has been carefully designed to provide an up-to-date, easy-to-understand, and reliable overview of the nursing procedures and principles most likely to be tested on the NCLEX-RN, and to furnish the graduate with the knowledge and confidence needed to excel on the licensure examination. It prepares the graduate for success in 3 important ways.

First, it reinforces the graduate's knowledge of the subject matter with carefully chosen questions and rationales in a written practice test, and with 100 additional questions on an interactive software computer disk with answers and rationales. All questions follow the latest NCLEX-RN test plan and format. Answers and rationales are given at the end of each chapter and are designed to teach the graduate *why* the correct answer is right and *why* the 3 distractors are incorrect.

All phases of the Nursing Process (Assessing, Planning, Implementing, and Evaluating) are identified for every question, as are Client Needs (Health Promotion and Maintenance, Physiological Integrity, Psychosocial Integrity, and Safe, Effective Care Environment). Graduates can easily trace their level of preparation in all of these areas.

Second, this practice test and review gives each graduate an opportunity to practice and learn the test-taking skills and strategies that are vital for success on the NCLEX-RN CAT. Practicing how to select correct answers using the Critical Thinking Process can improve test scores. Graduates who possess good test-taking skills and who are able to apply knowledge correctly are more likely to experience success on the NCLEX-RN.

Third, this review decreases test-taking anxiety. Many graduates tell us they study the material for tests but are so anxious they are unable to remember the subject matter being tested. This practice test and review increases confidence because it enables graduates to prepare appropriately and effectively and provides a quick and efficient way to assure success on the NCLEX-RN.

Directory of State and Territorial Boards of Registered Nursing

ALABAMA
Executive Officer
Alabama Board of Nursing
P.O. Box 303900
Montgomery, AL 36130-3900
Phone: (334) 242-4060

ALASKA
Executive Administrator
Alaska Board of Nursing
3601 C Street, Suite 722
Anchorage, AK 99503
Phone: (907) 269-8161

AMERICAN SAMOA
Executive Secretary
Pago Pago Health Services Regulatory Board
LBJ Tropical Medical Center
Pago Pago, AS 96799
Phone: (684) 633-1222

ARIZONA
Executive Director
Arizona State Board of Nursing
1651 East Morton, Suite 150
Phoenix, AZ 85020
Phone: (602) 255-5092

ARKANSAS
Executive Director
Arkansas State Board of Nursing
1123 South University, Suite 800
Little Rock, AR 72204
Phone: (501) 686-2700

CALIFORNIA
Executive Officer
Board of Registered Nursing
P.O. Box 944210
Sacramento, CA 94244-2100
Phone: (213) 897-3590

COLORADO
Program Administrator
Colorado State Board of Nursing
1560 Broadway, Suite 670
Denver, CO 82002-2410
Phone: (303) 894-2430

CONNECTICUT
Executive Officer
Department of Public Health-MS #12 NUR
Connecticut Board of Examiners for Nursing
410 Capitol Avenue
P.O. Box 340308
Hartford, CT 06134-0308
Phone: (860) 509-7624

DELAWARE
Executive Director
Delaware Board of Nursing
Cannon Building
P.O. Box 1401, Suite 203
Dover, DE 19901
Phone: (302) 739-4522, ext. 217

DISTRICT OF COLUMBIA
Contact Representative
District of Columbia Board of Nursing
614 H Street, N.W.
Washington, DC 20013
Phone: (202) 727-7856

FLORIDA
Executive Director
Florida State Board of Nursing
4080 Woodcock Drive, Suite 202
Jacksonville, FL 32207
Phone: (904) 858-6940

GEORGIA
Executive Director
Georgia Board of Nursing
166 Pryor Street, S.W.
Atlanta, GA 30334
Phone: (404) 656-5167

GUAM

Executive Director
Guam Board of Nurse Examiners
P.O. Box 2816
Agana, GU 96910
Phone: (671) 734-7295

HAWAII

Executive Officer
Hawaii Board of Nursing, Box 3469
Honolulu, HI 99503
Phone: (808) 586-2695

IDAHO

Assistant Executive Director
Idaho State Board of Nursing
P.O. Box 83720
Boise, ID 83720-0061
Phone: (208) 334-3110

ILLINOIS

Acting Coordinator
Illinois Department of Professional Regulation
320 West Washington Street
Springfield, IL 62786
Phone: (217) 785-9465

INDIANA

Director
Indiana State Board of Nursing
402 West Washington Street, Room W 041
Indianapolis, IN 46204
Phone: (317) 233-4405

IOWA

Executive Director
Iowa State Board of Nursing
1223 East Court Avenue
Des Moines, IA 50319-0166
Phone: (515) 281-4828

KANSAS

Executive Administrator
Kansas State Board of Nursing
900 S.W. Jackson Street, Suite 551-S
Topeka, KS 66612-1256
Phone: (913) 296-3782

KENTUCKY

Executive Director
Kentucky Board of Nursing
312 Whittington Parkway, Suite 300
Louisville, KY 40222-5172
Phone: (502) 329-7000, ext. 235

LOUISIANA

Executive Director
Louisiana State Board of Nursing
3510 N. Causeway Boulevard, Suite 501
Metairie, LA 70002
Phone: (504) 838-5332

MAINE

Executive Director
Maine State Board of Nursing
35 Anthony Avenue
State House Station #158
Augusta, ME 04333-0158
Phone: (207) 287-1133

MARYLAND

Executive Director
Maryland State Board of Nursing
4140 Patterson Avenue
Baltimore, MD 21215-2254
Phone: (410) 764-5142

MASSACHUSETTS

Executive Director
Board of Registration in Nursing
100 Cambridge Street, Room 150
Boston, MA 02202
Phone: (617) 727-3060

MICHIGAN

Nurse Consultant
Michigan Board of Nursing
P.O. Box 30018
611 West Ottawa
Lansing, MI 48909
Phone: (517) 373-4674

MINNESOTA

Executive Director
Minnesota Board of Nursing
2700 University Avenue, West #108
St. Paul, MN 55114
Phone: (612) 643-2565

MISSISSIPPI
Associate Commissioner
Institute of Higher Learning
3825 Ridgewood Road
Jackson, MS 39211
Phone: (601) 982-6690

MISSOURI
Executive Director
Missouri State Board of Nursing
3605 Missouri Boulevard, Box 656
Jefferson City, MO 65102-0656
Phone: (573) 751-0681

MONTANA
Executive Director
Montana State Board of Nursing
Arcade Building
111 North Jackson
Helena, MT 59620-0513
Phone: (406) 444-2071

NEBRASKA
Associate Director
Bureau of Examining Board
P.O. Box 95007
Lincoln, NE 68509
Phone: (402) 471-4917

NEVADA
Executive Director
Nevada State Board of Nursing
4335 South Industrial Road, #420
Las Vegas, NV 89103
Phone: (702) 739-1575

NEW HAMPSHIRE
Executive Director
State Board of Nursing
Division of Public Health
6 Hazen Drive
Concord, NH 03301
Phone: (603) 271-2323

NEW JERSEY
Executive Director
New Jersey Board of Nursing
P.O. Box 45010
Newark, NJ 07101
Phone: (201) 504-6499

NEW MEXICO
Executive Director
New Mexico Board of Nursing
4206 Louisiana Boulevard N.E., Suite A
Albuquerque, NM 87109
Phone: (505) 841-8340

NEW YORK
Executive Secretary
New York State Board of Nursing
The Cultural Center, Room 3023
Albany, NY 12230
Phone: (518) 486-2967

NORTH CAROLINA
Executive Director
North Carolina Board of Nursing
P.O. Box 2129
Raleigh, NC 27602
Phone: (919) 782-3211

NORTH DAKOTA
Executive Director
North Dakota Board of Nursing
919 South 7th Street, Suite 504
Bismarck, ND 58504-5881
Phone: (701) 328-9777

OHIO
Executive Director
Ohio Board of Nursing
77 South High Street, 17th Floor
Columbus, OH 43266-0316
Phone: (614) 466-9800

OKLAHOMA
Executive Director
Oklahoma Board of Nursing
2915 North Classen Boulevard, Suite 524
Oklahoma City, OK 73106
Phone: (405) 525-2076

OREGON
Executive Director
Oregon State Board of Nursing
800 N.E. Oregon Street, #25
Portland, OR 97232
Phone: (503) 731-4745

PENNSYLVANIA
Executive Secretary
Pennsylvania State Board of Nurses
P.O. Box 2649
Harrisburg, PA 17105
Phone: (717) 783-7142

PUERTO RICO
Acting Director
Council on Education
P.O. Box 19900 F. Juncos Station
San Juan, PR 00910-1900
Phone: (787) 724-7100

RHODE ISLAND
Director
Board of Nursing Education and
    Nurse Registration
Three Capitol Hill
Providence, RI 02908-5097
Phone: (401) 277-2827

SOUTH CAROLINA
Interim Program Manager
State Board of Nursing for South Carolina
220 Executive Center Drive, Suite 220
Columbia, SC 29210
Phone: (803) 896-4550

SOUTH DAKOTA
Education Specialist
South Dakota Board of Nursing
3307 South Lincoln Avenue
Sioux Falls, SD 57105
Phone: (605) 367-5940

TENNESSEE
Executive Director
Tennessee State Board of Nursing
283 Plus Park Boulevard
Nashville, TN 37217
Phone: (615) 532-5166

TEXAS
Executive Director
Texas Board of Nurse Examiners
Box 140466
333 Guadalupe 3-460
Austin, TX 78714
Phone: (512) 305-6818

UTAH
Executive Administrator
Utah State Board of Nursing
160 East 300 South, Box 45805
Salt Lake City, UT 84145
Phone: (801) 530-6628

VERMONT
Executive Director
Vermont State Board of Nursing
    Licensing and Registration Division
109 State Street
Montpelier, VT 05602
Phone: (802) 828-2396

VIRGIN ISLANDS
Executive Secretary
Virgin Islands Board of Nurse Licensure
P.O. Box 4247
Charolotte Amalie, VI 00803
Phone: (809) 776-7397

VIRGINIA
Executive Director
Virginia State Board of Nursing
6606 West Broad Street, 4th Floor
Richmond, VA 23230-1717
Phone: (804) 662-9951

WASHINGTON
Executive Director
Washington State Nursing Care Quality
    Assurance Commission
1300 Quince
P.O. Box 47864
Olympia, WA 98504-7864
Phone: (360) 664-4208

WEST VIRGINIA
Executive Secretary
West Virginia State Board of Registered
    Professional Nurses
101 Dee Drive
Charleston, WV 25311-1620
Phone: (304) 558-3596

WISCONSIN
Administrative Officer
Wisconsin Department of Regulation
    and Licensing
P.O. Box 8935
Madison, WI 53708-8935
Phone: (608) 267-2357

WYOMING
Executive Director
Wyoming State Board of Nursing
2301 Central Avenue
Barrett Building
Cheyenne, WY 82002
Phone: (307) 777-6127

Practice Test 1

Cardiocirculatory and Peripheral Circulatory Systems

1 - 1

A client is admitted to the Coronary Care Unit complaining of chest pain and nausea. Six hours after admission, the client tells the nurse, "I need to have a bowel movement." The most appropriate response by the nurse would be:

1. "You need to walk slowly to the bathroom. I will assist you."
2. "I will see that a commode chair is brought to your bedside."
3. "You should avoid straining while having a bowel movement."
4. "Wait until a prescription can be obtained for a fleet enema."

1 - 2

A client is admitted to the Intensive Cardiac Care Unit (ICCU) with a diagnosis of super-ventricular tachycardia. The client complains of dizziness and fatigue. In the presence of a rapid heart rate, the nurse will assess the client first for the development of:

1. fluid in the lungs.
2. pallor.
3. increasing urinary output.
4. unstable angina.

1 - 3

Your client is hypertensive and has been taking an angiotensin-converting enzyme inhibitor for several days. Today's medication prescriptions include the addition of a loop diuretic. The expected outcome of this therapy is:

1. excretion of calcium with no diuretic effect.
2. an increase in diastolic blood pressure.
3. a decrease in blood pressure.
4. hypotension.

1 - 4

A client diagnosed with acute myocardial infarction develops acute pericarditis 4 days after admission to the hospital. Nursing assessment on the fifth day of hospitalization reveals client complaints of chest pressure, shortness of breath, increasing anxiety, and restlessness. Physical findings show diminished heart sounds and a mild friction rub. The nurse recognizes these symptoms as evidence of:

1. cardiac tamponade.
2. pericardial effusion.
3. increased cardiac output.
4. cardiomyopathy.

1 - 5

Your client is unresponsive and has a pulse that is barely palpable. The electrocardiogram has identified a supraventricular tachycardia of 180 beats per minute (BPM). You will anticipate cardioversion by defibrillation with:

1. 200 joules.
2. 20 joules.
3. 50 joules.
4. 500 joules.

1 - 6

Isoxsuprine hydrochloride has been administered for a client with cerebrovascular insufficiency. The nurse can evaluate the effectiveness of this medication by:

1. monitoring vital signs frequently.
2. using the Doppler to assess peripheral pulses.
3. observing for an increased level of client activity.
4. determining the serum blood level of the drug.

1 - 7

A client with generalized arteriosclerosis approaches the nurse and says, "I don't sleep well at night because my feet get cold. What should I do?" Which of the following responses by the nurse would be most appropriate?

1. "Rub your feet briskly to improve circulation."
2. "Place a light blanket over your feet at night."
3. "Place your feet on a covered hot-water bottle."
4. "Put a covered heating pad on your feet with the dial on the lowest setting."

1 - 8

A client with esophageal varices is experiencing hematemesis. A balloon tamponade has been inserted. The nurse recognizes that the primary purpose of this intervention is to:

1. apply pressure to the affected area.
2. prevent paralytic ileus.
3. provide a means for irrigating the stomach.
4. prevent vomiting of blood.

1 - 9

A 3-year-old was hospitalized with congestive heart failure. The child has been digitalized and is now receiving a maintenance dose of digoxin 0.08 mg po bid. The available medication contains 0.05 mg digoxin per 1 cc of solution. How much of the solution will the nurse administer?

1. 0.06 cc
2. 0.6 cc
3. 1.6 cc
4. 2.6 cc

1 - 1 0

The most distinctive electrocardiogram change associated with hyperkalemia is:

1. absence of P waves.
2. atrial fibrillation.
3. heightened QRS complexes.
4. peaked T waves.

1 - 1 1

Which assessment should be completed frequently on clients receiving Tridil?

1. blood pressure
2. blood glucose
3. breath sounds
4. urine output

1 - 1 2

Atrial flutter may best be described as:

1. an irregular, chaotic ventricular rhythm.
2. an irregular rhythm with little wave formation between QRS complexes.
3. an atrial rhythm characterized by a sawtooth pattern between QRS complexes.
4. a barely discernible rhythm, not associated with heart muscle activity.

1 - 1 3

A client is receiving a continuous drip of nitroprusside sodium (Nipride) to decrease cardiac afterload. What special preparation will the nurse make when administering this medication?

1. Use special intravenous tubing.
2. Protect the solution from light.
3. Put the medication in glass bottles only.
4. Do not allow the solution to hang for more than 4 hours.

1 - 1 4

Your client has an asymptomatic abdominal aortic aneurysm. Ultrasonographic exam-ination indicates the aneurysm is 3.5 cm. You anticipate:

1. administration of an antihypertensive medication.
2. excision of the aneurysm and replacement of the excised segment with a synthetic graft.
3. a gastrointestinal bleed that may progress to shock.
4. a complaint by the client of intense back and flank pain with awareness of a pulsating mass in the abdomen.

1 - 1 5

You are concerned that your client is getting too much digoxin. What signs and symptoms are indicative of digitalis toxicity?

1. convulsions
2. yellow vision
3. muscle cramping
4. orthostatic hypotension

1 - 1 6

The nurse routinely obtains a client's central venous pressure readings. Should interven-tions become necessary based on the central venous pressure readings, they would be implemented for the purpose of:

1. maintaining a normal range of pressure in the right atrium.
2. lowering pressure in the pulmonary artery.
3. detecting dysrhythmias in the left ventricle.
4. promoting circulation through the aorta.

1 - 1 7

A client is diagnosed with Raynaud's phenomenon. When assisting the client to manage activities of daily living, the nurse should include which of the following in the teaching plan?

1. Move to a warmer climate.
2. Take pain medication when exposed to cold or cold objects.
3. Wear gloves when exposed to cold or cold objects.
4. Limit activity to decrease metabolic demands upon the body.

1 - 1 8

The foot of your client's casted leg is mottled and warmer than that of the unaffected leg. You notify the physician immediately because you suspect:

1. arterial insufficiency.
2. venous insufficiency.
3. compartmental syndrome.
4. fat emboli.

1 - 1 9

Which of the following symptoms is characteristic of intermittent claudication?

1. extensive discoloration
2. dependent edema
3. pain associated with activity
4. petechiae

1 - 2 0

A client experiencing stage II hypertension may be treated with which of the following medications?

1. levothyroxine
2. phenytoin
3. cefprozil
4. metroprolol

1-21

Your client has thromboangiitis obliterans. You are teaching the client how to participate in the treatment of this condition. Which statement by the client indicates a need for further teaching?

1. "It will be helpful if I can find employment that allows me to sit most of the time."
2. "I know it's essential that I quit smoking."
3. "I intend to walk 30 minutes twice daily."
4. "I'll need to be careful that I don't injure my legs."

1-22

The nurse is observing a client for symptoms of postoperative shock. The earliest symptom of postoperative shock would be obtained by monitoring the:

1. pulse rate.
2. pulse pressure.
3. temperature.
4. respirations.

1-23

A client with hypertension is receiving the angiotensin-converting enzyme inhibitor enalapril to decrease blood pressure. The nurse understands that this medication lowers blood pressure by:

1. promoting vasodilation.
2. blocking beta-adrenergic impulses.
3. inhibiting angiotensin-converting enzyme.
4. preventing reabsorption of sodium chloride.

1-24

A 65-year-old takes 0.125 mg of digoxin po qid. Which condition could predispose the client to develop digitalis toxicity?

1. pneumonia
2. hyperkalemia
3. hypothyroidism
4. hypocalcemia

1 - 2 5

A client complaining with severe substernal pain is presently being seen in the Emergency Department. An acute anterior myocardial infarction is suspected. An elevation of which enzyme would confirm the diagnosis at this time?

1. creatine kinase (CK) and its isoenzyme (CK-MB)
2. creatine kinase (CK) and its isoenzyme (CK-MM)
3. lactic dehydrogenase (LDH2)
4. serum glutamic-oxaloacetic transaminase

1 - 2 6

Which of the following laboratory value combinations is most likely to be representative of the client with the least risk of heart disease?

1. a high-density lipoprotein of 70 mg/dL and a low-density lipoprotein of 110 mg/dL
2. a high-density lipoprotein of 30 mg/dL and a low-density lipoprotein of 110 mg/dL
3. a high-density lipoprotein of 30 mg/dL and a low-density lipoprotein of 140 mg/dL
4. a high-density lipoprotein of 70 mg/dL and a low-density lipoprotein of 140 mg/dL

1 - 2 7

Your client is experiencing an evolving myocardial infarction and is being evaluated for thrombolytic therapy. Which statement made by the client would constitute a possible contradiction for this treatment?

1. "I've been having chest pain for 2 hours."
2. "I feel really nauseated right now."
3. "I've been taking blood pressure medicine for years."
4. "I'm still taking medicine for my stomach ulcers."

1 - 2 8

A client experiencing coronary artery disease may be treated with all of the following medications. Which medication will the nurse recognize as a calcium channel blocker?

1. metroprolol
2. nifedipine
3. nitroglycerin
4. aspirin

1 - 2 9

A 7-month-old infant with tetralogy of Fallot is in the recovery room following a right-heart catheterization. Which of the following assessment findings should be reported immediately?

1. an apical pulse of 74 beats per minute
2. the left foot is cool to the touch
3. mild clubbing of fingers and toes
4. irritable when dressing is changed

1 - 3 0

A client is returned to the unit following an angiocardiography. Which nursing action is appropriate at this time?

1. Discourage fluid intake and place the client in a prone position.
2. Apply heat to the puncture site and passively exercise the involved extremity.
3. Limit motion of the affected extremity and assess the puncture site.
4. Restrict fluid intake and encourage ambulation.

1 - 3 1

An adult client was admitted to the coronary care unit following a subendocardial myocardial infarction. A balloon-tipped pulmonary artery catheter was inserted when the client began to exhibit signs of cardiogenic shock. The nurse measures the client's pulmonary capillary wedge pressure and finds it to be 18 mm Hg. The nurse know this pressure is:

1. within normal limits.
2. elevated above normal.
3. less than normal.
4. life threatening.

1 - 3 2

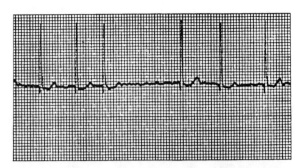

Your client's cardiac monitor displayed the above dysrhythmia. The client's blood pressure is 110/70 mm Hg, the pulse rate is 120/140 beats per minute, and the respiratory rate is 18 breaths per minute. The client is alert and oriented and complaining of palpitations and fatigue. The nurse will anticipate the administration of:

1. lidocaine.
2. atropine.
3. digitalis.
4. pronestyl.

1 - 3 3

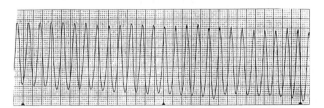

A 64-year-old client in the Intensive Coronary Care Unit is experiencing the above dysrhythmia. The client is hemodynamically stable. You will anticipate the administration of:

1. digoxin.
2. inderal.
3. lidocaine.
4. verapamil.

1-34

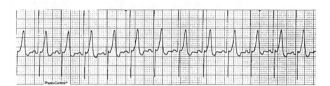

The nurse will recognize the above rhythm strip as an example of:

1. normal sinus rhythm.
2. sinus tachycardia.
3. ventricular tachycardia.
4. atrial fibrillation.

1-35

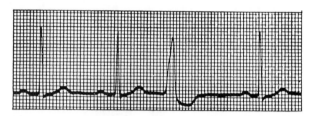

The above rhythm strip is an example of:

1. second-degree AV block, type II.
2. premature junctional contractions.
3. premature ventricular contractions.
4. third-degree AV block.

1-36

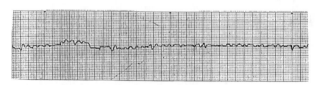

A client in the Intensive Coronary Care Unit converts to the above dysrhythmia. What should be done immediately?

1. cardioversion
2. defibrillation
3. administration of lidocaine
4. administration of sodium bicarbonate

1 - 3 7

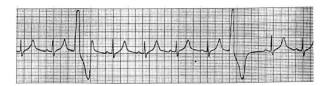

The above rhythm strip is an example of:

1. premature atrial contractions.
2. premature junctional contractions.
3. premature ventricular contractions.
4. third-degree AV heart block.

1 - 3 8

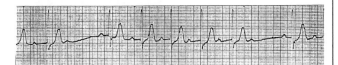

The above rhythm is an example of which dysrhythmia?

1. first-degree AV heart block
2. second-degree AV heart block, type I
3. second-degree AV heart block, type II
4. third-degree AV heart block

1 - 3 9

Sinus tachycardia may best be described by which of the following?

1. a chaotic rhythm with no discernible pattern and no cardiac output
2. a regular rhythm with a rate greater than 100 beats per minute
3. a ventricular rapid rhythm that may or may not produce a palpable pulse
4. a regular rhythm with rates between 60 and 100 beats per minute

1 - 4 0

Sinus bradycardia is best described as:

1. an irregular rhythm of ventricular origin with faint, if any, palpable pulse.
2. an irregular, slow ventricular rate with variable numbers of P waves between complexes.
3. a normal rhythm with a rate of less than 60 beats per minute.
4. a normal rhythm with a rate of more than 100 beats per minute.

1 - 4 1

A client who is to have Nitrostat on hand for the treatment of angina should be given which of the following instructions?

1. "Keep your medication in the refrigerator at all times."
2. "Replace your tablets every 2 years."
3. "Swallow your pill with a big glass of water, not milk."
4. "If your angina is not relieved after 3 pills, come to the Emergency Department."

1 - 4 2

Nursing measures that include instructing clients in the prevention of coronary artery disease are referred to as:

1. primary interventions.
2. acute-care interventions.
3. secondary interventions.
4. tertiary interventions.

1 - 4 3

A client who is taking daily digoxin says to you, "I have been experiencing nausea." Upon further inquiry, it is discovered that the client's pulse rate is 52 beats per minute. You should instruct the client to:

1. double the digoxin dose.
2. take an antacid 1 hour prior to today's digoxin dose.
3. take the digoxin on an empty stomach, but with a full glass of water.
4. hold the digoxin dose and come into the clinic for evaluation.

1 - 4 4

A client who has had a 12-lead electrocardiogram tells you there was a premature ventricular contraction noted by the technician taking the electrocardiogram. Your response to your client's concern about this is based on the knowledge that:

1. premature ventricular contractions may be benign.

2. there are no lifestyle changes that might decrease their incidence.

3. premature ventricular contractions are a prelude to lethal arrhythmias.

4. premature ventricular contractions indicate myocardial infarction.

Practice Test 1

Answers, Rationales, and Explanations

1 - 1

③ **The client should be told that straining at a stool is discouraged. Straining encourages the Valsalva's maneuver, which increases pressure in the large vein in the thorax and can interfere with the return of blood flow to the heart. The client should be provided with a bedpan to conserve energy.**

1. Clients admitted to a Coronary Care Unit (CCU) are placed on bed rest and should not walk to the bathroom.
2. Until a definitive diagnosis is made, the client should not use a bedside commode chair.
4. There is no indication that the client needs an enema.

Nursing Process: Implementing
Client Need: Health Promotion and Maintenance

1 - 2

① **The nurse will assess the client for the development of fluid in the lungs, which may be manifested by crackles (formerly referred to as rales). Rapid heart rhythms may cause heart failure along with accumulation of fluid in the lungs.**

2. Pallor (paleness of skin) may be present. However, the nurse will assess the client for the most life-threatening possibilities, such as fluid accumulation in the lungs.
3. Urinary output will be decreased in the presence of heart failure, not increased. Diminished cardiac output prevents an adequate supply of blood from reaching the body tissues and organs (low perfusion). Low perfusion of the kidneys causes an abnormal reduction in urinary output (oliguria).
4. Rapid heart rates are not always associated with unstable angina. However, fluid in the lungs is likely and life threatening.

Nursing Process: Assessing
Client Need: Physiological Integrity

1 - 3

③ **An expected outcome of loop diuretic therapy is a decrease in blood pressure. Loop diuretics are often administered with angiotensin-converting enzyme (ACE) inhibitors to manage hypertension. A diuretic reduces circulatory volume by increasing renal excretion of water, sodium, chloride, magnesium, hydrogen, and calcium. An ACE inhibitor prevents the production of angiotensin II, a potent vasoconstrictor. Therefore, by reducing circulatory volume and preventing vasoconstriction, the blood pressure can be lowered.**

1. When a loop diuretic is administered, it inhibits reabsorption (the absorbing of sodium and chloride by the nephron after they have passed through the glomerulus). The client will receive the benefit of the diuretic without the excretion of calcium.

2. Loop diuretics cause a decrease in diastolic blood pressure, not an increase.

4. Hypotension is a side effect of ACE inhibitors and diuretics, not an expected therapeutic outcome.

Nursing Process: Evaluating

Client Need: Health Promotion and Maintenance

1 - 4

② **Chest pressure, shortness of breath, anxiety, restlessness, diminished heart rate, and friction rub are all classic manifestations of pericardial effusion (the accumulation of an abnormally large amount of pericardial fluid in the pericardium).**

1. Cardiac tamponade may follow pericardial effusion. Symptoms of pericardial effusion include hypotension and elevated jugular vein distention (JVD).

3. Chest pressure, shortness of breath, anxiety, restlessness, diminished heart sounds, and friction rub would cause a decrease in cardiac output, not an increase in cardiac output.

4. Cardiomyopathy is a disease of the myocardium (the middle layer of the walls of the heart). Cardiomyopathy is characterized by impaired contractility and pumping ability of the heart.

Nursing Process: Analyzing

Client Need: Physiological Integrity

1 - 5

③ **Cardioversion by defibrillation with 50 joules is anticipated. Treatment for symptomatic supraventricular tachycardia is cardioversion. Defibrillation with 50 joules is the appropriate dosage.**

1. Defibrillation with 200 joules is indicated for ventricular fibrillation or pulseless ventricular tachycardia.
2. Defibrillation with 20 joules is a pediatric defibrillation dose.
4. Defibrillation with 500 joules is an inappropriate, excessive dosage of current.

Nursing Process: Planning
Client Need: Physiological Integrity

1 - 6

② **The effectiveness of isoxsuprine hydrochloride (Vasodilan) may be assessed by Doppler. Isoxsuprine hydrochloride (Vasodilan) is a beta-adrenerginic receptor stimulant whose impact on vascular smooth muscle causes vasodilation. Because of its vasodilatory effect, this medication is used to relieve the symptoms associated with conditions such as cerebrovascular insufficiency and peripheral vascular disease.**

1. The effectiveness of Vasodilan cannot be determined by monitoring the vital signs. Vital signs should be monitored to determine if the side effects of tachycardia and hypotension are present. Also, the client should be instructed to avoid sudden position changes because of the potential for orthostasis hypotension.
3. Vasodilan is not a stimulant. Therefore, the nurse will not expect an increase in client activity.
4. Serum blood levels for Vasodilan are not routinely monitored.

Nursing Process: Evaluating
Client Need: Health Promotion and Maintenance

1 - 7

② **The nurse should recommend that the client cover the feet with a light blanket. This is the most effective and safest way to keep the feet warm.**

1. Clients with arteriosclerosis are susceptible to thrombi formation. Therefore, rubbing the feet is dangerous since it could cause the release of thrombi.
3 and 4. Clients with poor circulation may experience paresthesia (numbness and tingling) of the extremities. For this reason, it would be unsafe to suggest the use of a hot-water bottle or a heating pad.

Nursing Process: Implementing
Client Need: Physiological Integrity

1 - 8

① **The primary purpose for the balloon tamponade is to apply pressure at the site of the bleeding esophageal varices. Esophageal varices are dilated, tortuous veins that may bleed easily. This condition is usually caused by portal hypertension and is life threatening.**

2. A paralytic ileus is characterized by lack of bowel sounds and lack of peristalsis accompanied by distention of the abdomen. The client may experience nausea and vomiting. Fecal material may be vomited because of the potential for reverse peristalsis. This condition is treated with a nasogastric tube, not a balloon tamponade. Paralytic ileus may occur following abdominal surgery or with the administration of certain psychotropic drugs.

3. Balloon tamponade does allow for gastric suctioning. However, this is not the primary purpose. Gastric suctioning is usually done to monitor bleeding.

4. Balloon tamponade will not prevent vomiting of blood. However, to prevent the aspiration of blood, an endotracheal tube is sometimes inserted.

Nursing Process: Evaluating
Client Need: Physiological Integrity

1 - 9

③ **The nurse will administer 1.6 cc of the solution. The following equation may be used:**

$$\frac{0.05\,mg}{1\,cc} = \frac{0.08\,mg}{X\,cc}$$

$$0.05X = 0.08$$

$$X = \frac{0.08}{0.05} = 1.6\,cc.$$

1, 2, and 4. All are incorrect dosages.

1 - 1 0

④ **The most distinctive electrocardiogram (ECG) change associated with hyperkalemia is an elevated T wave.**

1. The P wave represents atrial muscle depolarization. Absence of the P wave is associated with conditions such as atrial flutter and ventricular fibrillation.

2. Atrial fibrillation is a dysrhythmia in which minute areas of the atrial myocardium are in uncoordinated stages of depolarization and repolarization. This is due to multiple reentry circuits within the atrial myocardium. When this occurs, the atria quivers continuously in a chaotic pattern.

3. Heightened QRS complexes are associated with ventricular hypertrophy. Ventricular hypertrophy is due to chronic pressure overload.

Nursing Process: Evaluating
Client Need: Physiological Integrity

1 - 11

① **Clients receiving nitroglycerin (Tridil) intravenously should have their blood pressure monitored frequently. Tridil is the intravenous form of nitroglycerin. Because of its vasodilating effects, the blood pressure should be monitored frequently for the frequent side effect of hypotension.**

2. The administration of Tridil does not affect blood glucose.

3. The respiratory system is not directly affected by the administration of Tridil.

4. The genitourinary system is not directly affected by the administration of Tridil.

Nursing Process: Assessing

Client Need: Health Promotion and Maintenance

1 - 12

③ **Atrial flutter is best described as an atrial rhythm characterized by a sawtooth pattern between QRS complexes. Atrial flutter occurs when the sino-atrial node is no longer the primary atrial pacemaker and an ectopic pacemaker resumes pacing. This ectopic pacemaker may have a very high rate, which is represented as a sawtooth pattern on the electrocardiogram (ECG). The QRS complexes appear normal.**

1. An atrial flutter is not a ventricular rhythm.

2. An atrial flutter has a very definite pattern between the QRS complexes.

4. An atrial flutter is associated with heart muscle activity and there is a discernible rhythm.

Nursing Process: Assessing

Client Need: Health Promotion and Maintenance

1 - 13

② **When administering nitroprusside sodium (Nipride), the nurse will need to protect the fluid from light by wrapping the infusion bottle in aluminum foil. Nipride is a potent arterial/venous vasodilator that increases or decreases cardiac output depending on the extent of preload and afterload reduction.**

1. Unlike Tridil, Nipride does not require special intravenous tubing. However, Nipride should be mixed only with distilled water.

3. Unlike Tridil, Nipride does not require a glass bottle.

4. Nipride should not be left hanging for more than 24 hours.

Nursing Process: Planning

Client Need: Physiological Integrity

1 - 1 4

(1) **The nurse will anticipate administering an antihypertensive medication and scheduling ultrasonographic examinations every 6 months to determine any changes in the size of the aneurysm.**

2. Surgery is not generally performed when an abdominal aortic aneurysm is less than 4 to 5 cm.

3. Gastrointestinal bleeding that produces shock is the presenting sign when an abdominal aortic aneurysm ruptures into the duodenum.

4. Clients do not have complaints if their abdominal aortic aneurysm is asymptomatic.

Nursing Process: Planning

Client Need: Health Promotion and Maintenance

1 - 1 5

(2) **Signs and symptoms of digitalis toxicity include headaches, yellow vision, blurred vision, drowsiness, restlessness, muscle weakness, anorexia, nausea, vomiting, diarrhea, and cardiac dysrhythmias.**

1. Convulsions are not among the side effects of digoxin administration.

3. Muscle cramps are not among the side effects of digoxin administration.

4. Orthostatic hypotension is not among the side effects of digoxin administration. However, antihypertensive agents may cause orthostatic hypotension.

Nursing Process: Analyzing

Client Need: Physiological Integrity

1 - 1 6

(1) **The goal of any interventions based on central venous pressure (CVP) readings would be maintaining normal pressure in the right atrium. The CVP is an estimate of the pressure within the right atrium and provides information concerning the function of the right side of the heart. Changes in CVP represent changes in blood volume and in the venous return to the right side of the heart.**

2. Central venous pressure (CVP) readings estimate the pressure in the right atrium. CVP does not pertain to pressure in the pulmonary artery.

3. Central venous pressure (CVP) readings will not detect dysrhythmias in the left ventricle.

4. Central venous pressure (CVP) readings will not promote circulation through the aorta.

Nursing Process: Evaluating

Client Need: Physiological Integrity

1-17

③ **The nurse would recommend that the client who is experiencing Raynaud's phenomenon wear gloves when exposed to cold or cold objects. Raynaud's phenomenon is initiated by exposure to cold. (Occasionally it is initiated by emotional disturbance.) Raynaud's phenomenon is characterized by intermittent attacks of pallor followed by cyanosis, then the digits become red and return to normal.**

1. Moving to a warmer climate, although desirable, may not be beneficial since symptoms may continue to occur in the cooler weather of that climate.

2. Taking analgesics is not considered an activity of daily living.

4. Raynaud's phenomenon is a vasospastic disorder of small cutaneous arteries that is self-limiting. Episodes last only about 15 minutes, frequently involving the fingers. Limiting activities is not necessary.

Nursing Process: Planning
Client Need: Health Promotion and Maintenance

1-18

② **The nurse will suspect venous insufficiency and will notify the physician. With venous insufficiency, the casted limb feels warmer than the uncasted limb and appears bluish or mottled in color.**

1. The hallmark of arterial insufficiency is intermittent claudication, which is experienced as sharp, unrelenting, constant pain.

3. Compartmental syndrome occurs when a structure such as a nerve or tendon is constricted in a space, as in carpal tunnel syndrome. Symptoms include throbbing pain out of proportion to the original condition or injury, pain that is not relieved by analgesics, pain experienced when flexing or extending the affected body part.

4. A fat embolus produces symptoms that include hypoxia, tachycardia, dyspnea, and pallor.

Nursing Process: Analyzing
Client Need: Safe, Effective Care Environment

1-19

③ **Pain associated with activity is characteristic of intermittent claudication. The pain is caused by inadequate arterial circulation to contracting muscle. Severe pain occurs when walking and subsides with rest. The inadequate blood supply may be due to arterial spasms, atherosclerosis, arteriosclerosis, or an occlusion.**

1, 2, and 4. Extensive discoloration, dependent edema, and petechia are not characteristic of intermittent claudication.

Nursing Process: Analyzing
Client Need: Physiological Integrity

1 - 2 0

④ **A client with stage II hypertension may be treated with metroprolol (Lopressor). Metroprolol inhibits a portion of the sympathetic nervous system and reduces myocardial contractility, heart rate, and blood pressure. This medication belongs in the group of medications called beta blockers that are used to treat hypertension and arrhythmias. Stage II hypertension is hypertension with blood pressures of 160-170 mm Hg systolic and 100-109 mm Hg diastolic. These pressures are typically treated medically.**

1. Levothyroxine (Synthroid) is a thyroid hormone replacement and has no impact on hypertension.

2. Phenytoin (Dilantin) is an anticonvulsant and has no impact on hypertension.

3. Cefprozil (Cefzil) is an antibiotic and has no impact on hypertension.

Nursing Process: Implementing

Client Need: Physiological Integrity

1 - 2 1

① **The nurse will teach the client that sitting or standing in one position for long periods is not recommended since this contributes to venous stasis. Thromboangiitis obliterans (Buerger's disease) is characterized by inflammation of the small and intermediate arteries and veins. It results in the formation of thrombi and eventually in occlusion of vessels.**

2. Clients with Buerger's disease should absolutely not use tobacco in any form. Research indicates that heavy smoking is either a causative or a contributive factor. Cigarette smoking causes arterial constriction and increases platelet adhesion, which leads to thrombus formation.

3. Walking is advisable and helps prevent stasis of blood flow.

4. Clients with Buerger's disease should avoid injury to the extremities because of the likelihood of infection due to poor circulation.

Nursing Process: Implementing

Client Need: Health Promotion and Maintenance

1-22

① **The nurse would monitor the client's pulse rate for signs of postoperative shock. The earliest sign of shock is a pulse rate that steadily increases over time. An increase in the heart rate is an attempt to compensate for a decrease in cardiac volume.**

2. Pulse pressure is the difference between the diastolic and systolic pressures. The pulse pressure would drop if a client was in shock. However, a drop in pulse pressure would not be the earliest sign of shock.

3. Body temperature refers to the balance between the heat produced by the body and the heat lost by the body. A drop in body temperature would not be the first sign of shock.

4. Respiration would increase in response to postoperative shock, but this would not be the first sign of shock.

Nursing Process: Assessing
Client Need: Health Promotion and Maintenance

1-23

③ **Ace inhibitors such as enalapril (Vasotec) decrease blood pressure by inhibiting the angiotensin-converting enzyme. Therefore, angiotensin (a potent vasoconstrictor) is not released.**

1. Vasodilators such as hydralazine hydrochloride (Apresoline) and diazoxide (Hyperstat) act primarily on the smooth muscle of arterioles to cause vasodilation.

2. Beta-adrenergic blockers such as propranolol hydrochloride (Inderal) decrease blood pressure by blocking the beta-adrenergic impulses.

4. Diuretics such as furosemide (Lasix) block the reabsorption of sodium and chloride and thus decrease fluid volume and blood pressure.

Nursing Process: Evaluating
Client Need: Physiological Integrity

1-24

③ **Hypothyroidism affects the body's ability to metabolize digitalis and predisposes a client to digitalis toxicity.**

1. Pneumonia does not affect the body's ability to metabolize digoxin.

2. Hypokalemia, not hyperkalemia, predisposes a client to digitalis toxicity.

4. Hypercalcemia, not hypocalcemia, predisposes a client to digitalis toxicity.

Nursing Process: Evaluating
Client Need: Physiological Integrity

1 - 2 5

① An elevation of the CK (creatine kinase) MB (isoenzyme of creatine kinase associated with the cardiac muscle) is the best indication of myocardial damage within the first 2 to 4 hours following the acute ischemic event. The enzyme CK (MB) is found almost exclusively in the myocardium.

2. An elevation of CK (creatine kinase) MM (isoenzyme of creatine kinase associated with skeletal muscle) is an indicator of skeletal muscle damage, not myocardial damage.

3. An elevation of LDH_1 and LDH_2 is indicative of myocardial necrosis. Approximately 80% of clients show an increase of these enzymes within 48 hours after a myocardial infarction.

4. The enzyme SGOT (serum glutamic-oxaloacetic transaminase) is found in the liver, and to some extent, in the skeletal muscle. Therefore, an elevated SGOT is not helpful in confirming damage to the myocardium.

Nursing Process: Evaluating

Client Need: Physiological Integrity

1 - 2 6

① Laboratory values with the least risk for heart disease would be high-density lipoproteins (HDL) of 70 mg/dL and low-density lipoproteins (LDL) of 110 mg/dL. High-density lipoproteins, although a form of cholesterol, tend to bind with low-density lipoproteins, thereby lowering total cholesterol levels. HDL levels above 35 mg/dL are desirable. Low-density lipoproteins contribute to elevated total cholesterol levels, and levels <130 mg/dL are most desirable. The combination of an elevated HDL and low LDL will have the least risk for heart disease.

2, 3, and 4. All are associated with heart disease. An HDL of 30 mg/dL is too low and LDL levels >130 mg/dL are too high.

Nursing Process: Evaluating

Client Need: Health Promotion and Maintenance

1-27

④ Clients with stomach ulcers may not receive thrombolytic therapy. Thrombolytic therapy is the administration of medications specifically designed to dissolve blood clots. Muscle damage associated with arterial blockage by blood clots can be completely avoided with these medications. Because these medications affect blood viscosity and clotting mechanisms, possible contradictions include disorders that are hemorrhagic in nature. Bleeding ulcers, recent surgeries, blood dyscrasias, and aneurysms are examples of disorders that may constitute a contradiction for such treatment.

1. Antithrombolytic therapy has been found to be very successful if administered early in the course of the event.

2. Nausea is not an uncommon symptom associated with an evolving myocardial infarction and would not prevent a client from receiving antithrombolytic therapy.

3. Persons who take antihypertensive medications may take thrombolytic therapy.

Nursing Process: Analyzing
Client Need: Physiological Integrity

1-28

② Nifedipine (Procardia) is a calcium channel blocker. Calcium channel blockers tend to inhibit the flow of calcium ions across cell membranes. This class of drugs is specific for cardiac tissue and decreases excitability of cardiac tissue. As a result, the heart rate decreases and blood pressure drops.

1. Metroprolol (Lopressor) belongs in the group of drugs called beta blockers.

3. Nitroglycerin (Nitrostat) is an antianginal vasodilatory medication.

4. Aspirin is an antipyretic analgesic with antiplatelet activity.

Nursing Process: Evaluating
Client Need: Safe, Effective Care Environment

1-29

① An apical pulse of 74 beats per minute (BPM) is too low for an infant 7 months old and should be reported immediately. Cardiac catheterization can result in dysrhythmia or rates that are too slow or too fast. This may occur because of temporary or permanent damage to the conduction system.

2. Access to the vessels would have been in the right femoral area. Coolness of the left foot is most likely related to environmental temperature, not the catheterization.

3. Clubbing is not related to catheterization. It is related to the cardiac defect and usually develops slowly as a result of hypoxia to the distal tissues.

4. An 7-month-old infant may experience anxiety in the presence of strangers and in connection with a new procedure.

Nursing Process: Assessing
Client Need: Health Promotion and Maintenance

1-30

③ **The nurse will limit the motion of the affected extremity and assess the puncture site. The client is at risk for hemorrhage from the puncture site following an angiocardiography.**

1. Fluid intake should be encouraged to flush out the radiopaque dye used in the angiocardiography. However, the client should be placed in a supine position with the affected leg straight and the head elevated no more than 30 degrees.

2. Application of heat would facilitate hemorrhage, as would passive exercise to the affected extremity.

4. The client should be encouraged to drink plenty of fluids to flush out the dye used in the angiocardiography. Ambulation is contraindicated due to the likelihood of hemorrhage at the puncture site. The site needs time to heal.

Nursing Process: Implementing

Client Need: Health Promotion and Maintenance

1-31

② **The nurse will recognize a capillary wedge pressure of 18 mm Hg as elevated. The normal pulmonary capillary wedge pressure is 5 to 12 mm Hg. The higher the pressure, the more severe the heart failure. Pressures that exceed 25 to 30 mm Hg are associated with pulmonary edema.**

1. This client's pulmonary capillary wedge pressure is 18 mm Hg (normal is 5 to 12 mm Hg).

3. The capillary wedge pressure is above normal, not less than normal.

4. At this point, the pulmonary capillary wedge pressure is 18 mm Hg and is considered elevated. If the pressure should continue to rise, it would become life threatening.

Nursing Process: Analyzing

Client Need: Physiological Integrity

1-32

③ **The nurse will anticipate the administration of digitalis. The rhythm shown on the client's monitor depicts atrial fibrillation. It is characterized by an irregular rhythm with no identifiable P waves.**

1. Lidocaine (Xylocaine) is administered to treat ventricular tachycardia.

2. Atropine (Atropair) increases the heart rate. Therefore, it would not be administered since the client's heart rate is already fluctuating between 120 to140 beats per minute (BPM). Atropine is administered to clients who have slow rhythms.

4. Procainamide (Pronestyl) is frequently indicated for ventricular dysrhythmia, not atrial dysrhythmia.

Nursing Process: Planning

Client Need: Physiological Integrity

1 - 3 3

③ **Lidocaine (Xylocaine) is the drug of choice for clients who experience ventricular tachycardia and are hemodynamically stable.**

1. Digoxin (Lanoxin) is the drug of choice for atrial fibrillation.

2 and 4. Propranolol (Inderal) and verapamil (Calan) are administered for supraventricular tachycardia.

Nursing Process: Planning
Client Need: Physiological Integrity

1 - 3 4

② **The nurse will recognize the rhythm strip as an example of sinus tachycardia. There is a P wave for every QRS, the rhythm is regular, and the PR interval and QRS intervals are within normal limits. The only abnormality is the rate.**

1. The rate of a normal sinus rhythm is between 60 and 100 beats per minute (BPM). Sinus tachycardia has a rate between 100 and 150 BPM.

3. Ventricular tachycardia is characterized by 3 or 4 consecutive premature ventricular contractions.

4. Atrial fibrillation is characterized by an irregular rhythm with no identifiable P wave.

Nursing Process: Assessing
Client Need: Physiological Integrity

1 - 3 5

③ **The rhythm strip is an example of premature ventricular contractions. The PVCs are characterized by wide, bizarre QRSs, no associated P waves preceding the QRS complex, and T waves in the opposite direction from the QRS deflection.**

1. Second-degree A V block type II results in intermittently dropped QRS complexes with normal-appearing P waves occurring at regular intervals.

2. Premature junctional contractions are characterized by upward impulses from the A V junction to the atria; thus in lead II the P waves are inverted and the PR interval shortens to 0.12 seconds.

4. In third-degree A V block, all impulses from the atria are blocked, resulting in complete disassociation of the atria and ventricles and causing differences in heart rate and QRS durations.

Nursing Process: Assessing
Client Need: Physiological Integrity

1 - 3 6

② **The immediate treatment is defibrillation. The dysrhythmia depicted is ventricular fibrillation. This is characterized by a bumpy line of unidentifiable waves. This is a life-threatening dysrhythmia and without prompt treatment death will occur.**

1. Cardioversion cannot be performed because cardioversion requires that the electric shock be correlated with the QRS complex. There are no QRS complexes with ventricular fibrillation. The machine will never fire if it is programmed for cardioversion.

3. Lidocaine (Xylocaine) is utilized for ventricular tachycardia and frequent PVCs. After defibrillation and restoration of a rhythm, a lidocaine drip will probably be initiated to decrease the irritability of the myocardium, but first the rhythm must be converted out of ventricular fibrillation.

4. Sodium bicarbonate is administered to correct the acidosis that occurs with the arrest situation. It will probably be given to a client with ventricular fibrillation, but again, the client needs to be defibrillated first. If the client is not converted, the client will die.

Nursing Process: Implementing
Client Need: Physiological Integrity

1 - 3 7

③ **The rhythm strip depicts unifocal premature ventricular contractions. PVCs are characterized by wide, bizarre QRSs, no associated P waves preceding the QRS complex, and T waves in the opposite direction from the main QRS deflection.**

1. Premature atrial contractions are characterized by a premature P wave with a contour different from that of a sinus P wave. The QRS complex may or may not be normal, and the premature beat is followed by a pause approximately equal to the sinus cycle.

2. Premature junctional contractions will have P waves that are inverted, premature, and precede the QRS complex; or the P wave may be hidden in the QRS or inverted and following the QRS. The QRS is normal, but the PR interval is less than 0.12 seconds.

4. With third-degree A V block, the atria and ventricles beat independently, and there is no association between the atria and the ventricles.

Nursing Process: Analyzing
Client Need: Physiological Integrity

1 - 3 8

② **This strip depicts second-degree A V block, type I. This dysrhythmia is characterized by a PR interval that progressively lengthens until a P wave is not followed by a QRS complex.**

1. First-degree A V block is characterized by a PR interval greater than 0.20 seconds.

3. Second-degree A V block, type II is characterized by nonconducted sinus impulses despite constant PR intervals.

4. In third-degree A V block, all the sinus or atrial impulses are blocked and the atria and ventricles are forced to beat independently.

Nursing Process: Analyzing

Client Need: Physiological Integrity

1 - 3 9

② **Sinus tachycardia may best be described as a regular rhythm with a rate greater than 100 beats per minute. Sinus tachycardia is defined as a rhythm that originates in the sinus node and follows the normal conduction pathways through the ventricles. In the adult client, the parameters of sinus tachycardia are generally considered to be 100 to 150 beats per minute (BPM). Rates of greater than 150 beats per minute are not thought to originate from the sinoatrial node, but from an ectopic site above the ventricles; hence the term "supraventricular tachycardia."**

1. Chaotic rhythm with no cardiac output is most likely a ventricular fibrillation.

3. A ventricular rhythm with variable output is most likely ventricular tachycardia.

4. A regular rhythm with rates between 60 and 100 beats per minute is usually considered to be normal sinus rhythm in the adult client.

Nursing Process: Analyzing

Client Need: Physiological Integrity

1 - 4 0

③ **Sinus bradycardia is best described as a normal rhythm with a rate of less than 60 beats per minute (BPM). Sinus bradycardia is defined as a rhythm that originates from the sinus node and follows the regular conduction pathways through the ventricles. In the adult client, rates of less than 60 beats per minute (BPM) are considered to be bradycardic. This term does not define a pathology; it defines a rhythm that may be completely benign.**

1. An irregular ventricular rhythm would describe an idioventricular or ventricular rhythm.

2. An irregular ventricular rate with variable numbers of P waves between complexes describes a complete or third-degree heart block.

4. A normal rhythm with a rate of greater than 100 BPM describes sinus tachycardia.

Nursing Process: Analyzing

Client Need: Physiological Integrity

1 - 4 1

④ **As a rule, chest pains that are not relieved by 3 doses of nitroglycerin should be evaluated by a physician. Anginal pain is often managed well and without complications. However, angina which is not relieved by repeated doses of nitroglycerin should be evaluated for myocardial ischemia or infarction.**

1. Nitroglycerin should be kept with the client who experiences angina and should be accessible; protecting the medication from extreme temperatures is usually adequate for storage.

2. Nitroglycerin is usually replaced ever 6 months to ensure freshness of the medication.

3. This medication is to be taken via the sublingual route, not swallowed.

Nursing Process: Implementing

Client Need: Physiological Integrity

1 - 4 2

① **Primary interventions are those that contribute to the prevention of a disease process. Examples of primary intervention include immunizations against disease and teaching wellness.**

2 and 3. Acute and secondary interventions focus on the diagnosis and treatment of a disease process.

4. Tertiary interventions focus on rehabilitation from a disease process.

Nursing Process: Implementing

Client Need: Health Promotion and Maintenance

1 - 4 3

④ **Clients who experience nausea and have a pulse rate of 52 beats per minute (BPM) should be instructed to withhold their morning dose of digoxin and come to the office or hospital for evaluation. Digoxin is a cardiac antiarrhythmic with positive inotropic qualities (it regulates and strengthens the heart's contractions). Digoxin toxicity is a risk for anyone taking this medication, however, because it has a relatively narrow therapeutic range. Signs and symptoms of digoxin toxicity include nausea, dizziness, visual disturbances, bradycardias, or other arrhythmias.**

1. This client may be experiencing digoxin toxicity. Therefore the client should not be advised to take more digoxin until further evaluation.

2. Antacids are not recommended in this situation because they could mask symptoms.

3. When digoxin is taken, it is recommended that it be taken on an empty stomach.

Nursing Process: Implementing

Client Need: Physiological Integrity

1 - 4 4

(1) **Premature ventricular contractions (PVCs) may be benign contractions that originate from the ventricles, rather than the atria, and are early in the cycle. They are usually wide and rather bizarre in their morphology. It is not uncommon to notice rare PVCs on a monitored client who has no cardiac pathology; they may be completely benign.**

2. PVCs may be caused by substances that increase sympathetic tone, such as caffeine and nicotine.

3. They do not necessarily indicate a pending lethal arrhythmia, although frequent premature ventricular contractions, symptomatic PVCs, or coupled PVCs may indicate an arrhythmia disorder.

4. Clients experiencing myocardial infarctions may have numerous arrhythmias, including PVCs; however, all persons having PVCs are not necessarily experiencing a myocardial infarction.

Nursing Process: Evaluating

Client Need: Physiological Integrity

Practice Test 2

Endocrine System and Diabetes

2 - 1

An emaciated client is to receive NPH insulin 20 units 1 hour before breakfast daily. The insulin should be administered:

1. intramuscularly at 90 degrees.
2. subcutaneously at 90 degrees.
3. intramuscularly at 45 degrees.
4. subcutaneously at 45 degrees.

2 - 2

An adolescent 15 years of age is hospitalized with Type I insulin–dependent diabetes. Which of the following is essential to teach the client?

1. Insulin dosage will be determined by food intake.
2. Insulin will have to be administered the rest of the client's life.
3. Insulin dosage will be adjusted by the way the client eats.
4. Insulin will be adjusted as the client grows older.

2 - 3

A client's insulin is to be given intravenously. Which insulin will you administer?

1. Regular
2. NPH
3. Ultralente
4. Lente

2 - 4

Your client is receiving 30 units of NPH insulin each morning at 7:00 a.m. What would the client need to do each day?

1. exercise for 30 minutes prior to lunch
2. consume a snack each day at 4:00 p.m.
3. exercise for 30 minutes prior to bedtime
4. consume a bedtime snack at 9:00 p.m.

2 - 5

A 26-year-old gravida I has Type I insulin-dependent diabetes. Due to a change in insulin requirements during the first trimester, the nurse will carefully observe the client for signs of:

1. hypoglycemia.
2. ketoacidosis.
3. hyperglycemia.
4. pregnancy-induced hypertension.

2 - 6

A client is to receive 12 units of Regular insulin and 26 units of NPH insulin subcutaneously daily. Which procedure is correct?

1. Store all insulin in the refrigerator.
2. Massage the injection site after the injection.
3. Draw up the NPH insulin first, and then the Regular.
4. Roll the NPH insulin bottle between the palms of the hands prior to drawing up the dose.

2 - 7

Your client was started on 0.1 mg of Synthroid daily. What teaching will the client need in relation to this medication?

1. Take medication with meals.
2. Do not substitute generic brands.
3. Dosage can be self-adjusted based on energy needs.
4. Expect to lose 10 to 15 pounds within the first 6 months of therapy.

2 - 8

Your client had a bilateral adrenalectomy and Solu-Cortef has been prescribed. You know the purpose of this medication is to:

1. lower serum glucose.
2. relieve postoperative pain.
3. prevent adrenal insufficiency.
4. decrease the risk of postoperative stress ulcers.

2 - 9

A 22-year-old female is admitted to the unit with a blood glucose of 822 mg/dL and an arterial blood pH of 7.02. The client is unresponsive. The insulin type and route you anticipate is:

1. Humulin N given intravenously.
2. Humulin R given intravenously.
3. Humulin 70/30 given intravenously.
4. Humulin N given subcutaneously only.

2 - 1 0

A client is admitted to the nursing unit with a medical diagnosis of chronic hypothyroidism. The nursing assessment reveals a body temperature of 90° F, an apical heart rate of 58, and a respiratory rate of 10 per minute. The nurse immediately recognizes these findings as indicative of:

1. hypercalcemia.
2. hypermagnesemia.
3. metabolic acidosis.
4. myxedema coma.

2 - 1 1

A client with diabetes has been taking tolazamide 100 mg po daily. The client has just had a hip replacement and is to be on coumadin 5 mg po daily. You anticipate the following potential changes:

1. an increase in serum glucose levels.
2. a decrease in prothrombin times.
3. a decrease in serum glucose and an increase in prothrombin times.
4. an increase in serum glucose and an increase in prothrombin times.

2 - 1 2

A client arrives in the Emergency Department restless, hypotensive, confused, and vomiting. The client's friend states that the client stopped taking betamethasone 4 days ago because it tended to cause heartburn. You anticipate the administration of:

1. large doses of loop diuretics.
2. narcotic analgesics.
3. sodium bicarbonate and Humulin N intravenously.
4. glucocorticoids.

2-13

Your client is being treated with glucocorticoids for adrenal insufficiency secondary to abrupt withdrawal of cortisone. Your client's friend asks you what happened to the client's adrenal glands. You explain that:

1. the adrenal glands were destroyed by the cortisone therapy.
2. the adrenal glands were not really affected and "adrenal insufficiency" is just a loosely applied term.
3. the adrenal glands have probably developed tumors.
4. the adrenal function was suppressed during the cortisone therapy.

2-14

Your client has been placed on a regime of methylprednisolone because of severe allergies. Your client teaching will include instructions to:

1. taper the medication dose according to the regime.
2. take the medication only on days when allergies flare up.
3. discontinue taking the medication when the symptoms of allergies are no longer noticeable.
4. contact the physician because this is not a recommended therapy for allergic reactions.

2-15

During a thyroidectomy, a client's parathyroid glands were inadvertently removed. Which of the following laboratory tests must be monitored very closely?

1. urine specific gravity
2. creatine kinase-MB isoenzyme
3. serum calcium
4. amylase

2-16

The nurse recognizes that clients receiving large dosages of vasopressin may experience:

1. facial pallor.
2. headache.
3. flushing.
4. dyspnea.

2-17

An adolescent with diabetes asks about the use of alcohol. The most appropriate counsel would be:

1. Diabetics require more insulin when they consume alcohol.
2. Alcohol consumption increases blood glucose.
3. Hypoglycemia occurs with alcohol consumption.
4. Diabetics who consume alcohol become intoxicated easily.

2-18

The physician prescribed 20 units of isophane (NPH) insulin 30 minutes before breakfast daily for a client with diabetes mellitus. The client is to have a midafternoon snack of milk and crackers. The client asks the nurse why the snack is necessary. Which response by the nurse would be best?

1. "It will improve your nutritional status."
2. "It will improve carbohydrate metabolism."
3. "It prevents an insulin reaction."
4. "It prevents diabetic ketoacidosis."

2-19

A client with hypoparathyroidism complains of tingling of the lips, hands, and face. You notify the physician because you suspect the development of which complication?

1. syndrome of inappropriate antidiuretic hormone
2. tetany
3. myxedema
4. Cushing's syndrome

2-20

Hyperthyroidism is suspected in a 28-year-old client. Prescriptions include a radioactive iodine uptake test. The nurse will explain to the client that the chief purpose of a radioactive iodine uptake test is to:

1. ascertain the ability of the thyroid gland to produce thyroxine.
2. measure the activity of the thyroid gland.
3. estimate the concentration of thyrotropic hormone in the thyroid gland.
4. determine the best method of treating the thyroid condition.

2-21

A client develops carpopedal spasms subsequent to a subtotal thyroidectomy. Which of the following medications will the nurse have available for administration?

1. calcium gluconate
2. potassium chloride
3. diazepam
4. phenytoin sodium

2-22

A client undergoes a subtotal thyroidectomy. During the immediate postoperative period, the nurse should assess for laryngeal nerve damage. Which of the following findings would indicate the presence of this problem?

1. facial twitching
2. wheezing
3. hoarseness
4. hemorrhage

2-23

Which laboratory value should be monitored closely in a client with hypoparathyroidism?

1. calcium
2. sodium
3. potassium
4. cholesterol

2-24

An insulin-dependent diabetic is scheduled for surgery. Administration of Regular insulin is prescribed in lieu of isophane insulin. The client asks why the insulin prescription had to be changed. Which explanation by the nurse would be best?

1. Stress-induced fluctuations in blood glucose can be more adequately managed with Regular insulin.
2. During the first week following recovery from diabetic acidosis, the likelihood of a recurrence is greatest.
3. Diminished activity intensifies the body's response to long-acting insulin.
4. Diabetic acidosis causes a temporary increase in the rate of food absorption.

2-25

A mother makes all of the following comments about her 3-month-old infant daughter to the nurse. Which comment will indicate to the nurse that the infant may have thyroid hormone deficiency?

1. "My baby smiles a lot."
2. "My baby's good and never cries."
3. "My baby notices toys and knows my voice."
4. "My baby spends a great deal of time watching her hands."

2-26

The physician has prescribed warm saline dressings to be applied to a heel ulcer of a diabetic client. You observe another nurse preparing a clean basin and washcloth to implement the procedure. Which of the following actions should you take?

1. Interrupt the nurse assembling supplies to discuss the procedure.
2. Present the situation for discussion at a staff meeting.
3. Do nothing, as the nurse is following the correct procedure.
4. Do nothing, because nurses are accountable for their own actions.

2-27

A client with Addison's disease is admitted to your unit. What do you expect your assessment to reveal?

1. osteoporosis
2. hirsutism
3. sodium and water retention
4. dark pigmentation of skin

2-28

A client with noninsulin-dependent diabetes mellitus takes 5 mg po daily of glyburide for glucose control. Which statement by the client indicates a need for further teaching?

1. "I will not take an extra pill if I eat too much."
2. "I will eat 3 meals a day."
3. "I will call my physician if I get sick."
4. "I will take my pill every night before I go to bed."

2-29

The physician has written the following prescriptions for a client with myxedema. Which prescription will you question?

1. levothyroxine sodium 0.2 mg intravenously every day
2. nitroglycerin gr 1/150 sublingually prn for chest pain
3. morphine sulfate 4 mg intravenously every 4 hours prn for severe pain
4. monitor capillary blood glucose at 7:00 a.m., 11:00 a.m., 4:00 p.m., and 9:00 p.m.

2-30

A client had a subtotal thyroidectomy. While assessing, the nurse observes that the client swallows frequently and speaks with a twang. The blood pressure is 20 points lower, the pulse is 30 points higher, and respirations are twice as fast than baseline admission assessment. Which of the following is an appropriate nursing action?

1. Continue to monitor vital signs every 30 minutes as prescribed.
2. Record findings; considering the client's postoperative state, vital signs are within normal ranges.
3. Notify the surgeon; the client may be bleeding internally.
4. Report findings to the nursing supervisor.

2-31

A client with myxedema was admitted to your unit. What do you expect your assessment to reveal?

1. weight loss
2. subnormal temperature
3. tachycardia
4. hirsutism

2-32

You are planning a teaching program for a 16-year-old who has recently been diagnosed with Type I diabetes. When planning the program, you understand the greatest influence on its success is:

1. the client's acceptance of the diagnosis.
2. the parents' acceptance of the diagnosis.
3. whether or not the entire teaching plan is implemented by the same nurse.
4. whether or not teaching is limited to 1-hour periods.

2 - 3 3

A mother with diabetes mellitus has delivered her baby. Two hours after delivery, the nurse observes that the infant is lethargic and has developed mild generalized cyanosis and twitching. The nurse should recognize that the infant is probably exhibiting symptoms of:

1. hypoglycemia.
2. hypercapnia.
3. hypothermia.
4. hypercalcemia.

2 - 3 4

Which of the following measures is the most effective in achieving normal blood sugar levels in the client with Type II diabetes?

1. increasing sodium intake
2. decreasing water intake
3. achieving ideal body weight
4. decreasing daily exercise

2 - 3 5

Your client has a closed head injury and is experiencing increased intracranial pressure. You will monitor the client for potential damage to the:

1. adrenal gland.
2. parathyroid gland.
3. thyroid gland.
4. pituitary gland.

2 - 3 6

Acromegaly is due to:

1. undersecretion of the thyroid hormones.
2. oversecretion of the growth hormone.
3. absence of the sex hormones.
4. undersecretion of the antidiuretic hormone.

2-37

Increased levels of serum calcium may result in which of the following?

1. increased secretion of growth hormone
2. increased secretion of parathormone
3. decreased secretion of follicle-stimulating hormone
4. decreased secretion of parathormone

2-38

Clients experiencing hypothyroidism are generally treated with thyroid replacement therapy. Which of the following is a potentially serious side effect of the initiation of thyroid replacement?

1. angina
2. increased urination
3. increase in energy level
4. myxedema

2-39

A client is to receive Lugol's solution 0.2 ml tid 12 days prior to a thyroidectomy. The nurse knows to administer this medication:

1. on an empty stomach.
2. immediately before meals.
3. diluted in juice and taken through a straw.
4. with an iodine-rich food.

2-40

An infant is receiving levothyroxine for the treatment of congenital hypothyroidism. The infant's parents should be taught to notify their child's health-care provider if they observe:

1. mottled and cool skin.
2. a pulse rate above 150 beats per minute.
3. feeding difficulty.
4. edema and weight gain.

2-41

The following diagnostic studies have been prescribed: protein-bound iodine, radioactive iodine uptake, and triiodothyronine. Which of the following instructions will the nurse give to prepare the client for these procedures?

1. Food and fluids are restricted prior to these procedures.
2. Proper imaging of the thyroid during these tests requires restricting movement.
3. The tests may take some time because injected dyes travel slowly to the thyroid.
4. Ingestion of iodine is restricted prior to these tests.

2-42

A client has pheochromocytoma. The nurse will monitor the client's:

1. blood pressure.
2. respiratory rate.
3. hemoglobin level.
4. white blood cell count.

2-43

A client who is experiencing manifestations of a pituitary tumor will probably complain of:

1. decrease in peripheral vision.
2. tearing and eye pain with exposure to sunlight.
3. dependent edema.
4. dyspnea.

2-44

Which of the following medications would most likely be administered to treat the signs and symptoms associated with Graves' disease?

1. epinephrine
2. codeine
3. beta-blockers
4. laxatives

Practice Test 2

Answers, Rationales, and Explanations

2 - 1

④ Emaciated clients should have insulin administered at a 45-degree angle into the sub-cutaneous tissue. The first factor to consider is the emaciated state of this client. Because of the client's emaciated condition, the nurse will give the injection at a 45-degree angle.

1 and 3. Insulin is administered subcutaneously, not intramuscularly.

2. At a 90-degree angle, the injection would go through the subcutaneous tissue of an emaciated client.

Nursing Process: Implementing
Client Need: Physiological Integrity

2 - 2

② Exogenous insulin will need to be administered the rest of the client's life. Persons with Type I diabetes have little or no endogenous insulin.

1, 3, and 4. All are important facts regarding insulin dosage, but it is most essential for the adolescent to know insulin injections will be required throughout life.

Nursing Process: Implementing
Client Need: Physiological Integrity

2 - 3

① Regular insulin is the only insulin that can be given intravenously. Regular insulin is clear and does not contain any modifying agents.

2, 3, and 4. NPH, Ultralente, and Lente insulins contain modifying agents and cannot be administered intravenously.

Nursing Process: Analyzing
Client Need: Safe, Effective Care Environment

2 - 4

② Since NPH insulin peaks in 6 to 8 hours, the client should consume a snack at 4:00 p.m. to prevent hypoglycemia. The onset of NPH insulin is 2 hours, peak 6 to 8 hours, and duration 12 to 16 hours.

1 and 3. Daily exercise should be accounted for and adjustments in daily insulin dosages need to be made based on exercise regimens. Additional glucose needs to be consumed if the client exercises more than usual, since exercise has a hypoglycemic effect.

4. Long-acting insulin given at bedtime requires a bedtime snack the next day (onset 2 hours, peak 16 to 20 hours, duration 24+ hours).

Nursing Process: Planning

Client Need: Health Promotion and Maintenance

2 - 5

① The nurse will observe the client for signs of hypoglycemia. There is a decreased need for insulin in the first trimester. The level of human placental lactogen (HPL) (an insulin antagonist) is low. Also, the client and the developing fetus use more glucose and glycogen.

2 and 3. Ketoacidosis accompanies hyperglycemia, not hypoglycemia.

4. Pregnancy-induced hypertension is not a factor in the first trimester.

Nursing Process: Assessing

Client Need: Health Promotion and Maintenance

2 - 6

④ NPH insulin is an Intermediate-acting insulin. The bottle should be rolled between the palms of the hands to thoroughly mix the dose prior to withdrawal of the dose.

1. Insulin in use may be left at room temperature for up to 4 weeks unless the room temperature is higher than 85°F or below freezing. Extra insulin may be stored in the refrigerator.

2. After injecting insulin, some pressure should be applied to the site while the needle is being withdrawn. The swab should be held in place for a few seconds, but the site should not be massaged because massage may cause bruising.

3. When mixing an Intermediate-acting insulin with Regular insulin, the Regular insulin should always be drawn up first.

Nursing Process: Planning

Client Need: Health Promotion and Maintenance

2 - 7

② Clients receiving Synthroid (levothyroxine) should not substitute generic brands. Different brands of thyroid preparations may not be the same. To maintain appropriate thyroid levels, no substitutes are allowed.

1. Synthroid (levothyroxine) does not have to be taken with meals. However, it is recommended that it be taken at the same time each day to establish consistency.
3. The dosage of Synthroid cannot be self-adjusted. The dosage needs to be adjusted based on serum laboratory values and is adjusted only under the direction of a qualified health-care provider.
4. Weight loss may occur as a result of an increase in basal metabolic rate, but it may not occur for all clients.

Nursing Process: Implementing
Client Need: Safe, Effective Care Environment

2 - 8

③ Hydrocortisone (Solu-Cortef) will replace the corticosteriod normally produced in the adrenal gland's cortex and prevent adrenal insufficiency.

1. Solu-Cortef tends to raise serum glucose levels rather than lower them.
2. Solu-Cortef is not an analgesic and will not relieve postoperative pain.
4. Solu-Cortef causes gastric irritation and should be administered with meals.

Nursing Process: Evaluating
Client Need: Health Promotion and Maintenance

2 - 9

② You will anticipate administering Humulin R intravenously. Humulin R is a rapid-acting insulin and is administered to treat high blood glucose levels.

1. Humulin N is in suspension and cannot be given intravenously.
3. Humulin 70/30 insulin cannot be given intravenously. It is a combination of 70 units of Intermediate insulin and 30 units of Regular insulin.
4. A rapid-acting insulin is needed. Humulin N cannot be given intravenously.

Nursing Process: Planning
Client Need: Physiological Integrity

2-10

④ **The nurse will associate the client's symptoms with myxedema coma. A body temperature of 90°F, an apical heart rate of 58 beats per minute (BPM), and respirations of 10 per minute are classic symptoms of myxedema coma seen in clients who have hypothyroidism.**

1. Hypercalcemia (calcium serum levels above 10.1 mg/dL) may be seen in hyperthyroidism, not hypothyroidism.

2. Hypermagnesemia (magnesium serum levels above 2.1 mg/dL) is a condition associated with acute adrenocortical insufficiency and untreated diabetic ketoacidosis.

3. Symptoms of metabolic acidosis include increased respiratory rate and depth, not bradypnea (abnormally slow breathing).

Nursing Process: Assessing
Client Need: Physiological Integrity

2-11

③ **You will anticipate a decrease in serum glucose and an increase in prothrombin times. Tolazamide (Tolinase) and warfarin (Coumadin) tend to augment each other's actions. Therefore, the prothrombin time will increase and the serum glucose levels will be lowered even more since the two drugs are being used in combination.**

1. A combination of Tolinase and Coumadin tends to decrease serum glucose levels even more than when administering Tolinase alone.

2. A combination of Tolinase and Coumadin tends to increase the prothrombin time even more than when Coumadin is administered alone.

4. A combination of Tolinase and Coumadin tends to decrease serum glucose levels.

Nursing Process: Evaluating
Client Need: Health Promotion and Maintenance

2-12

④ **You will anticipate the administration of glucocorticoids. This person is exhibiting classic signs of adrenal insufficiency, probably due to the abrupt cessation of glucocorticoid therapy.**

1. Diuretics are usually not given to hypotensive clients because they lower blood pressure by decreasing circulating volume.

2. An analgesic is not anticipated since there is no indication that the client is experiencing pain.

3. There is no indication that the client is experiencing metabolic acidosis and would require sodium bicarbonate.

Nursing Process: Planning
Client Need: Physiological Integrity

2-13

④ **You will explain that the function of the adrenal glands is suppressed during glucocorticoid therapy and abrupt cessation of glucocorticoids does not allow time for the adrenal glands to resume normal functioning.**

1. There is no evidence of permanent adrenal damage.
2. The adrenal function was affected by glucocorticoid use.
3. There is no evidence of an adrenal tumor.

Nursing Process: Implementing

Client Need: Physiological Integrity

2-14

① **The client will be taught to taper the methylprednisolone (Medrol) according to the regime. Tapering the dosage will avoid adrenal insufficiency.**

2. Corticosteroids such as methylprednisolone (Medrol) are to be taken on a regular basis, not just when an allergy is bothersome.
3. Sudden withdrawal of a corticosteroid can precipitate adrenal insufficiency.
4. Methylprednisolone (Medrol) is an appropriate medication for the treatment of allergic reactions.

Nursing Process: Implementing

Client Need: Health Promotion and Maintenance

2-15

③ **Serum calcium should be monitored carefully. The parathyroid gland's function is to increase calcium absorption and increase blood calcium levels. Serum calcium levels must be scrupulously monitored. Extreme disturbances in calcium levels may lead to tetany or lethal arrhythmias.**

1. Urine specific gravity is not directly affected by parathormone (PTH).
2. Creatine kinase (CK) and its isoenzyme (CK-MB) are monitored to confirm an acute myocardial infarction. CK-MB is not associated with parathormone (PTH).
4. Amyalase is an enzyme associated with the pancreas, not the parathyroid gland.

Nursing Process: Evaluating

Client Need: Health Promotion and Maintenance

2 - 1 6

① **When large dosages of vasopressin (Pitressin) are administered, a client may experience facial pallor due to the drug's vasoconstrictive action.**

2. Clients may experience dizziness and a "pounding" sensation in the head, but not a headache.

3. Clients may experience perspiration, paleness, and perioral blanching, but not flushing.

4. Dyspnea is not associated with the administration of Pitressin.

Nursing Process: Assessing
Client Need: Physiological Integrity

2 - 1 7

③ **Diabetics should be taught that alcohol consumption inhibits the release of glycogen from the liver, which results in hypoglycemia.**

1 and 2. Alcohol does not increase the need for more insulin or increase the blood glucose level. However, it does inhibit the release of glycogen from the liver, which results in hypoglycemia.

4. Diabetics who drink alcohol do not become intoxicated any sooner or later than people who drink alcohol and don't have diabetes. However, diabetics may develop hypoglycemia and fail to get the proper medical help because their symptoms may appear to be those associated with alcohol intoxication.

Nursing Process: Evaluating
Client Need: Physiological Integrity

2 - 1 8

③ **Receiving a midafternoon snack will prevent an insulin reaction. Isophane insulin is an Intermediate-acting insulin with a peak action of 6 to 12 hours. During peak action time, maximum insulin effect is expected to occur. To prevent an insulin reaction, proper food supplements must be given.**

1. The snack of milk and crackers is given strictly to prevent an insulin reaction. It has nothing to do with improving the client's nutritional status.

2. The crackers are a source of carbohydrates that will prevent an insulin reaction and hypoglycemic rebound.

4. Diabetic ketoacidosis (DKA) is caused by an absence or insufficient amount of insulin.

Nursing Process: Implementing
Client Need: Health Promotion and Maintenance

2-19

②　The nurse will suspect the development of tetany. Hypoparathyroidism causes a decrease in serum calcium levels due to a lack of parathyroid hormone stimulation. A decrease in calcium ion concentration causes tetany. Signs of tetany syndrome include tingling of the lips, hands, and feet; muscle tension; stiffness; and paresthesia (sensation of numbness).

1. Syndrome of inappropriate antidiuretic hormone (SIADH) is a complication of conditions such as increased intracranial pressure (ICP) and endocrine and pulmonary disorders. It is associated with an increase in the secretion of antidiuretic hormone (ADH), which causes an extracellular volume overload and a decrease in urine output.

3. Myxedema is a type of hypothyroidism associated with the extreme symptoms of that condition.

4. Cushing's syndrome results from excessive adrenocortical activity, not hypoparathyroidism.

Nursing Process: Analyzing
Client Need: Physiological Integrity

2-20

②　The purpose of a radioactive iodine uptake test is to measure the activity of the thyroid gland. The thyroid gland cannot distinguish between regular iodine and radioactive iodine. By administering tracer doses of radioactive iodine and calculating the percentage of radioactive iodine used by the gland to produce thyroxine, gland activity can be measured. In clients with hyperthyroidism, the gland may use up to twice as much iodine as in a euthyroid (normal) state.

1. A radioactive iodine uptake test does not determine the ability of the thyroid gland to produce thyroxine.

3. A radioactive iodine uptake test does not estimate the concentration of thyrotropic hormone (thyroid-stimulating hormone) in the thyroid gland.

4. Treatment will not be addressed until a thorough assessment of the client has been completed. The radioactive iodine uptake test is only one consideration.

Nursing Process: Implementing
Client Need: Safe, Effective Care Environment

2-21

① **The nurse will have calcium gluconate available. When a client develops carpopedal spasms (spasms of the hands and feet) subsequent to a thyroidectomy, calcium gluconate should be administered. Muscular twitching and hyperirritability of the nervous system indicates tetany due to hypocalcemia. This condition develops if the parathyroid glands are accidentally removed during thyroid surgery. Calcium replacement therapy is indicated for the treatment of this problem.**

2. Potassium chloride (Slow-K) is administered for the treatment of potassium deficiencies and digitalis intoxication. It is not affected by a thyroidectomy.

3. Diazepam (Valium) is a sedative/hypnotic, anticonvulsant, and skeletal muscle relaxant. It does not replace calcium.

4. Phenytoin sodium (Dilantin) is an anticonvulsant and does not replace calcium.

Nursing Process: Planning

Client Need: Physiological Integrity

2-22

③ **Hoarseness and weakness of the voice following a subtotal thyroidectomy is an indication of laryngeal nerve damage. The damage occurs if there is unilateral injury of the pharyngeal nerve during surgery.**

1. Facial twitching may occur if the parathyroid glands are damaged or removed during the thyroidectomy.

2. Wheezing could occur as a result of edema, not laryngeal nerve damage.

4. Hemorrhage could occur following a thyroidectomy due to the vascularity of the operative site. However, hemorrhage would not indicate laryngeal nerve damage.

Nursing Process: Assessing

Client Need: Physiological Integrity

2-23

① **Clients with hypoparathyroidism should have their calcium level monitored closely. Hypoparathyroidism is characterized by hypocalcemia resulting from a lack of parathyroid hormone, which normally maintains serum calcium levels. Hypoparathyroidism may be caused by accidental removal or damage to the vascular supply of the parathyroid gland during surgery. As a consequence of hypocalcemia, tetany may develop. Signs of tetany include tingling of the lips, hands, and feet, progressing to muscle tension, paresthesias, and stiffness. The objective of treatment is to elevate the serum calcium level to 9 to 10 mg/dL.**

2, 3, and 4. Sodium, potassium, and cholesterol are not affected by hypoparathyroidism.

Nursing Process: Analyzing

Client Need: Physiological Integrity

2 - 2 4

① Stress-induced fluctuations in blood glucose can be more adequately managed with **Regular insulin. Regular insulin is rapid acting, beginning within 15 minutes after administration. It peaks within 2 to 4 hours and duration is 5 to 8 hours. Regular insulin is the only insulin that may be used intravenously when the client's blood glucose is out of control. Regular insulin may also be used with Intermediate or long-acting insulins to maintain better control. Regular insulin is the only insulin that can be used in the insulin pump. The use of Regular insulin with this client will minimize occurrence of intraoperative and postoperative complications associated with blood glucose levels.**

2. There is no indication that the client is or will be experiencing diabetic acidosis.

3. The long-acting insulin will not be used because it cannot be administered intravenously and is not fast acting. Regular insulin is needed to adequately manage blood glucose levels.

4. There is no indication that the client is experiencing diabetic acidosis. Also, food absorption is not affected by insulin.

Nursing Process: Implementing
Client Need: Physiological Integrity

2 - 2 5

② An early indication that the infant may have thyroid hormone deficiency is the statement by the mother, "My baby's good and never cries." Early manifestations of hypothyroidism are inactivity, excessive sleeping, and minimal crying, which leads a parent to the erroneous conclusion that a child is a quiet and good baby.

1, 3, and 4. A normal 3-month-old infant should be smiling, vocalizing, and noticing surroundings.

Nursing Process: Analyzing
Client Need: Physiological Integrity

2 - 2 6

① The nurse assembling the supplies should be interrupted and informed regarding the need for sterile technique. The client is a diabetic with a foot ulcer and is susceptible to infection and gangrene. Sterile technique is an essential factor in the client's recovery.

2. Presenting the situation for discussion at a staff meeting could jeopardize the client's health. Immediate action should be taken to prevent contamination of the client's foot ulcer.

3. Sterile technique is required when applying soaks to a foot ulcer of a client with diabetes.

4. Safe practice should be monitored by any nurse directly or indirectly involved in client care.

Nursing Process: Implementing
Client Need: Safe, Effective Care Environment

2-27

④ An assessment of a client with Addison's disease would reveal dark pigmentation of the skin, especially the sun-exposed areas over joints and creases such as the palms of the hands. Other assessment findings in the early period of the disease include muscular weakness, hypotension, fatigue, emaciation, anorexia, and low blood glucose. Addison's disease (adrenal insufficiency) results from a deficiency in the secretion of the adrenocortical hormones due to autoimmune influences (75% cases) and other conditions such as surgical removal, infection, or tuberculosis of the adrenal glands.

1. Adrenocortical insufficiency does not affect reduction in bone mass (osteoporosis).

2. Hirsutism (excessive growth of hair or presence of hair in unusual places) is not associated with adrenocortical insufficiency.

3. Sodium and water retention are not associated with adrenocortical insufficiency.

Nursing Process: Assessing
Client Need: Physiological Integrity

2-28

④ Clients who have noninsulin-dependent diabetes mellitus and are taking glyburide (Micronase) for glucose control should take the medication at the same time daily at breakfast or at the first main meal. Following administration, the medication is absorbed within 1 hour, peaks between 2 and 4 hours, and lasts 24 hours.

1. Glyburide (Micronase) po should be taken once daily. Extra doses are contraindicated.

2. Clients receiving glyburide (Micronase) should consume 3 meals a day on a regular schedule.

3. Clients receiving glyburide (Micronase) who become ill should notify the physician. It may be necessary to control blood glucose levels with Regular insulin administered intravenously.

Nursing Process: Implementing
Client Need: Health Promotion and Maintenance

2-29

③ The nurse will question a prescription for morphine sulfate. Clients who have myxedema (a type of hypothyroidism) are sensitive to sedatives, opiates, and anesthetic agents. The nurse should question any prescription for these medications.

1. Levothyroxine (Synthroid), a thyroid hormone replacement, is an appropriate medication.

2. Nitroglycerin is an appropriate medication since clients with myxedema are likely to have elevated serum cholesterol levels and coronary artery disease.

4. Monitoring capillary blood glucose is necessary since Synthroid increases the metabolic rate of body tissue.

Nursing Process: Analyzing
Client Need: Physiological Integrity

2-30

③ **The client's behavior and vital signs indicate internal bleeding and the surgeon should be notified. As a result of bleeding, tracheal narrowing has occurred, causing the client to speak with a nasal twang.**

1. Just monitoring the client's vital signs every 30 minutes is inadequate. The nurse must recognize that the client may be hemorrhaging and notify the surgeon.

2. The client's vital signs indicate changes beyond normal postoperative expectations.

4. The surgeon should be notified since internal bleeding is probable.

Nursing Process: Analyzing
Client Need: Physiological Integrity

2-31

② **The nurse would expect an assessment of a client with severe hypothyroidism (myxedema) to include a subnormal body temperature, bradycardia, and weight gain. The client's skin becomes thickened, the face expressionless, and mental processes are dulled. Early symptoms of myxedema include fatigue, hair loss, brittle nails, dry skin, numbness and tingling of fingers, and hoarseness.**

1. Weight gain would be expected in clients with myxedema (a type of hypothyroidism).

3. Bradycardia would be expected, not tachycardia.

4. Thinning and dryness of hair is associated with myxedema, not hirsutism (increased growth of hair or hair occurring in unusual places).

Nursing Process: Assessing
Client Need: Physiological Integrity

2-32

① **The nurse will recognize that the client's acceptance of the diagnosis will have the greatest influence on the success of the teaching program. In initiating a teaching plan, the nurse will be aware that the client is an adolescent in the process of forming a unique identity and accepting the self as a significant, capable person who is able to assume responsibility.**

2. The ultimate success of the program will depend on the client's acceptance of the diabetic condition, not the parents' acceptance of their child's condition. Adolescents are usually more concerned about what their peers' attitudes are, not what their parents think.

3. The number of health-care providers involved in the teaching plan should not affect its success.

4. Teaching should not exceed 1-hour periods. Clients who are learning about their condition, dietary restriction, and medication need time to absorb what is being taught.

Nursing Process: Planning
Client Need: Health Promotion and Maintenance

2 - 3 3

① **The nurse will recognize that the neonate of the diabetic mother is experiencing hypoglycemia. Prior to delivery, the fetus was exposed to high levels of maternal glucose. The fetus responded to the high glucose levels by increasing insulin production and hyperplasia of the pancreatic beta cells. Following the birth of the infant, the maternal glucose supply is gone and the infant becomes hypoglycemic as a result of high levels of circulating insulin.**

2. There is no reason to suspect hypercapnia (increased amounts of carbon dioxide serum levels). Hypercapnia is associated with conditions such as chronic obstructive pulmonary disease (COPD).

3. The cyanosis is due to hypoglycemia, not hypothermia.

4. Hypercalcemia (calcium serum levels above 10.0 mg/dL) is not associated with infants born of diabetic mothers.

Nursing Process: Analyzing

Client Need: Physiological Integrity

2 - 3 4

③ **Achieving ideal body weight is effective in maintaining normal blood sugar levels. The number of insulin receptors is decreased in the very obese. Many obese persons who experience marked fluctuations in their blood sugars find their blood sugars can be regulated with weight loss. Obese people tend to be insulin resistant.**

1. Increasing sodium in the diet may lead to hypertension and electrolyte imbalance.

2. Decreasing water intake may lead to dehydration.

4. Regular daily exercise is encouraged for clients who experience hyperglycemia. Exercise stimulates insulin production.

Nursing Process: Evaluating

Client Need: Health Promotion and Maintenance

2-35

④ A client experiencing a closed head injury should be monitored for evidence of damage to the pituitary gland, which is located on the inferior portion (base) of the brain. Pressure may be exerted on the pituitary gland if the brain swells. Fluctuations in blood pressure or diuresis may be evident in the client experiencing an increase in intracranial pressure because of the lack of vasopressin secreted by the pituitary gland. Although all endocrine function may be affected by a head injury, the pituitary gland is especially vulnerable due to the effects of increased intracranial pressure.

1. The adrenal glands are located near the kidneys.

2 and 3. Both the parathyroid glands and thyroid glands are located in the neck.

Nursing Process: Assessing
Client Need: Physiological Integrity

2-36

② Acromegaly, or enlargement of the viscera, develops as a result of oversecretion of growth hormone (GH). This hormone is secreted by the pituitary gland. Oversecretion of growth hormone in early childhood may result in giantism.

1, 3, and 4. Neither thyroid hormone, antidiuretic hormones, or sex hormones directly affect bone and viscera growth.

Nursing Process: Analyzing
Client Need: Physiological Integrity

2-37

④ Elevated serum calcium levels will result in decreased secretion of parathormone. Parathormone is the hormone secreted by the parathyroid glands. Parathormone regulates calcium metabolism and is affected by serum calcium levels. A feedback loop exists, as evidenced by a decrease in parathormone secretion with elevated serum calcium levels and vice versa.

1 and 3. Neither growth hormone nor follicle-stimulating hormone is directly affected by serum calcium levels.

2. An increase in serum calcium levels will result in a decrease in parathormone secretion.

Nursing Process: Analyzing
Client Need: Physiological Integrity

2-38

① **At the time thyroid replacement therapy is initiated, the client could experience the side effect of angina. Clients who experience hypothyroidism for extended periods have often developed elevated cholesterol levels and atherosclerotic changes in their vessels. They also tend to have a slow heart rate and relatively low metabolic demands. With the institution of thyroid replacement therapy, the metabolic rate increases, as does the heart rate. This may precipitate angina or an ischemic cardiac event.**

2. A marked increase in urination is not associated with instituting thyroid replacement therapy.

3. An increase in energy level is a desirable effect of thyroid replacement therapy.

4. Myxedema occurs as a result of hypothyroidism, not thyroid replacement therapy.

Nursing Process: Evaluating

Client Need: Health Promotion and Maintenance

2-39

③ **Lugol's solution should be diluted in fruit juice, water, or milk and taken through a straw. Iodine may cause nausea and vomiting and will also stain the teeth.**

1 and 2. Lugol's solution should be taken at meals to prevent gastric irritation.

4. Iodine-rich foods are not permitted because they interfere with the dosage of the prescribed iodine. High-iodine foods include iodized salts, oysters, spinach, lima beans, beef liver, and navy beans.

Nursing Process: Implementing

Client Need: Health Promotion and Maintenance

2-40

② **A pulse rate above 150 beats per minute (BPM) indicates possible tachycardia and can be a sign of too much levothyroxine.**

1, 3, and 4. Mottled and cool skin, feeding difficulty, edema, and weight gain are all signs of hypothyroidism and suggest that the medication level has not yet eliminated these symptoms.

Nursing Process: Evaluating

Client Need: Physiological Integrity

2-41

④ Ingestion of iodine is restricted prior to tests that utilize iodine. The protein-bound iodine (PBI) and the triiodothyronine (T-3) uptake tests are blood studies. The radioactive iodine uptake shows the percentage of radioactive iodine ingested orally that has been stored in the thyroid gland. No special preparation is needed for any of these tests. However, ingesting iodine in the form of iodized salt, foods, or drugs may alter the results of these tests.

1. There is no need to restrict food or fluids for any of these diagnostic studies.

2. There is no imaging required with any of these tests.

3. No dyes are injected. The client is given a po tracer dose of 131 iodine when preparing for the radioactive iodine uptake test.

Nursing Process: Implementing
Client Need: Safe, Effective Care Environment

2-42

① Clients with pheochromocytoma should have their blood pressure monitored closely. Pheochromocytoma is a tumor of the adrenal medulla. Functioning tumors of the adrenal medulla cause hypertension and other cardiovascular disturbances. Life-threatening blood pressures as high as 350/200 mm Hg have been recorded.

2, 3, and 4. Pheochromocytoma does not directly affect the client's respiratory rate, hemoglobin level, or white blood cell count.

Nursing Process: Implementing
Client Need: Physiological Integrity

2-43

① Clients who are experiencing manifestations of a pituitary tumor will probably complain of a decrease in peripheral vision. Complaints of visual field disturbance are not uncommon in clients with a pituitary tumor. Growing pituitary tumors may exert pressure on surrounding structures. Visual fields may be affected by the tumor's growth as pressure is exerted on the optic chiasm.

2. Tearing and eye pain with exposure to sunlight is often due to a disorder in the eye itself, such as increased pressure due to glaucoma.

3 and 4. Dyspnea and dependent edema are most likely due to disorders of the cardiovascular or renal systems, such as congestive heart failure, fluid overload, or respiratory disorders.

Nursing Process: Assessing
Client Need: Physiological Integrity

2 - 4 4

③ **Beta-blockers may be prescribed for clients with Graves' disease. Graves' disease (a form of hyperthyroidism) is associated with signs and symptoms of accelerated metabolism. Tachycardia, nervousness, and tremors are typical signs of this condition. Beta-blockers tend to slow the heart rate and are thus very useful in the adjunct therapy for Graves' disease.**

1. Epinephrine tends to increase, not decrease, the sympathetic nervous system response.

2. Codeine's analgesic effects are not indicated for this typically painless disease.

4. Laxatives are rarely indicated because persons with Graves' disease tend to have hyperactive bowel function.

Nursing Process: Evaluating

Client Need: Health Promotion and Maintenance

Practice Test 3

Gastrointestinal System and Nutrition

3 - 1

Your client is receiving continuous naso-gastric feedings. You know to change the tube feeding container and line every:

1. 8 hours.
2. 12 hours.
3. 24 hours.
4. 48 hours.

3 - 2

The most accurate assessment for correct placement of a nasogastric tube is to:

1. determine the pH of aspirate.
2. visualize the gastric area by X ray.
3. inject air into the tube and auscultate over the gastric area for the sound of air entering the stomach.
4. palpate the gastric area following the injection of 100 cc of air into the tube.

3 - 3

The nurse is discussing the treatment for gastroesophageal reflux with the parents of a newly diagnosed 4-month-old infant. Which comment by the parents indicates a need for more education?

1. "Our baby may develop pneumonia or breathing problems."
2. "Surgical correction will be needed when our baby is about 1 year of age."
3. "We may need to use formula thickened with rice cereal."
4. "We will try to feed more often and not as much at a time."

3 - 4

A client experiencing upper gastrointestinal bleeding was stabilized in the Emergency Department and was admitted to the hospital for further evaluation. To determine the cause and specific site of the bleeding, the nurse will anticipate a prescription for which diagnostic test first?

1. gastroscopy
2. gastrointestinal X rays
3. fiberoptic colonoscopy
4. gastric analysis

3 - 5

A client who is to be weighed daily on bed scales is receiving continuous liquid feedings via a percutaneous endoscopic gastrostomy. An important nursing intervention would be to:

1. weigh the day's feeding formula and add it to the client's weight.
2. inform the physician that persons receiving continuous feedings cannot be weighed on the bed scales.
3. defer the daily weighings and record this deferment on the chart.
4. turn the feedings off at least 30 minutes prior to the weighing process.

3 - 6

Your client had a resection of a diseased portion of the ileum. Which instruction will you give the client about performing deep breathing and coughing exercises?

1. "Sit in an upright position, take a deep breath, and then cough."
2. "Hold your abdomen firmly, take several deep breaths, and then cough 2 or 3 times as you exhale."
3. "Tighten your stomach muscles as you inhale and then cough forcefully."
4. "Raise your shoulders to expand your chest and then give a deep cough."

3 - 7

Ingestion of which of the following foods has been found to exacerbate gastro-esophageal reflux disease?

1. poultry
2. pastas
3. herbs and spices
4. caffeine and chocolate

3 - 8

A client is experiencing vomiting and gastro-intestinal bleeding. You are to prepare an intravenous infusion containing potassium chloride. The purpose of administering potassium chloride is to:

1. replace potassium that is lost in the urine.
2. restore lost potassium reserves.
3. provide potassium to promote excretion of sodium.
4. replace the potassium that is being lost through vomiting.

3 - 9

Your client had a subtotal gastrectomy and may experience the dumping syndrome as a direct result of:

1. the removal of a large portion of the stomach.
2. hyperosmolar chyme.
3. consuming large quantities of food.
4. not resting after each meal.

3 - 1 0

How many ounces a day of commercially prepared formula will contain 500 kcal of energy?

1. 5 ounces
2. 15 ounces
3. 25 ounces
4. 50 ounces

3 - 1 1

A 10-lb baby requires how many kilocalories per day for energy?

1. 100 kcal
2. 500 kcal
3. 1000 kcal
4. 1500 kcal

3 - 1 2

A client was admitted to the hospital with Crohn's disease. What do you expect your assessment to reveal?

1. diarrhea and abdominal pain
2. jaundice and steatorrhea
3. shortness of breath and tachycardia
4. dependent edema and ascites

3 - 1 3

Which of the following may result from prolonged gastroesophageal reflux disease and can quickly become life threatening?

1. pharyngitis
2. colitis
3. esophageal ulceration
4. angina

3 - 1 4

Which of the following diets would be the most appropriate for a client who has hyper-cholesterolemia?

1. hamburger patty, macaroni and cheese, iced tea
2. baked chicken breast, apple, skim milk
3. fish sticks, French fries, cola
4. pizza, tossed salad, beer

3 - 1 5

During a physical assessment, your client tells you, "I belch a lot and when I lie down undigested food comes up into my mouth. I have noticed a gurgling sound after eating, and I have a sour taste in my mouth." You suspect a:

1. diffuse esophageal spasm.
2. gastroesophageal reflux.
4. hiatal hernia.
5. pharyngoesophageal diverticulum.

3 - 1 6

Your client has a history of scarring as a result of repeated ulcerations and healings of ulcers distal to the pyloric sphincter. Recent complaints include epigastric fullness, pain, distention, nausea, vomiting, and anorexia. The client states that the pain is worse at night. You suspect:

1. peptic ulcer perforation.
2. acute gastritis.
3. pyloric obstruction.
4. paralytic ileus.

3 - 1 7

Your client is experiencing the acute phase of ulcerative colitis. The client states, "There is blood in my stools. I'm afraid." You will:

1. check the client's stools for the presence of occult blood.
2. recommend that the client keep a record of the number and description of stools.
3. notify the client's physician immediately.
4. explain to the client that blood in the stools is expected in this condition.

3 - 1 8

A client with cirrhosis of the liver has a serum bilirubin level of 50 mg/dL. In order to evaluate these laboratory results, you need to know that the normal serum bilirubin level is:

1. 0.2 to 1.0 mg/dL
2. 3 to 10 mg/dL
3. 10 to 20 mg/dL
4. 20 to 30 mg/dL

3 - 1 9

Your client will have a permanent colostomy following a colon resection. You will teach the client that the colostomy should begin to function postoperatively:

1. 12 to 24 hours.
2. 2 to 4 days.
3. 4 to 5 days.
4. 5 to 6 days.

3 - 2 0

A 4-year-old child is acutely ill. Which of the following nursing measures will be most helpful in meeting the child's nutritional needs during the acutely ill period?

1. serving foods that are lukewarm
2. giving liquids through a straw
3. offering small frequent feedings of favorite foods
4. allowing the client to select foods from the regularly scheduled meal trays

3 - 2 1

A client had an abdominoperineal resection with the creation of an end colostomy. A sump drain was left in the client's perineal wound. The purpose of the sump drain is to:

1. allow for easy assessment of the character and volume of the drainage.
2. allow for easy passage of flatus until peristalsis returns.
3. prevent contamination of the operative site secondary to frequent dressing changes.
4. allow wound healing from its lowest depth without forming an abscess.

3 - 2 2

A client asks, "Why am I receiving aluminum hydroxide?" You will explain that the expected action of this drug is to:

1. aid in inhibiting the secretion of hydrochloric acid.
2. serve as a catalyst in the breakdown of proteins.
3. absorb air that has been swallowed.
4. neutralize gastric secretions.

3 - 2 3

A 73-year-old client was admitted to the hospital with vomiting and gastrointestinal bleeding. The nurse prepares to administer an intravenous infusion that contains potassium chloride. The nurse will explain to the client that the purpose of the infusion is to:

1. replenish the potassium that is being lost in the urine.
2. replace the potassium that is lost through vomiting.
3. restore the potassium level that elderly clients cannot maintain through normal dietary intake.
4. provide potassium in an amount sufficient to promote excretion of sodium chloride.

3 - 2 4

You are encouraging an elderly client to increase intake of protein. To provide the greatest amount of protein you will plan to add which of the following to 100 cc of milk?

1. 50 cc of light cream and 2 tablespoons of corn syrup
2. 30 grams of powdered skim milk and 1 egg
3. 1 small scoop (90 grams) of vanilla ice cream and 1 tablespoon of chocolate syrup
4. 2 egg yolks and 1 tablespoon of sugar

3-25

You are preparing a client for an upper gastrointestinal series. Which of the following explanations by the nurse would be both accurate and appropriate to share with the client?

1. "In the X-ray Department, you will be asked to drink a thick liquid, and then several X rays of the upper part of your digestive system will be taken at intervals."

2. "You will be asked to swallow a tube so that your physician can look at the lining of your stomach. X rays will be taken at the same time."

3. "You will be asked to swallow a substance that is radioactive, and then a series of X rays will be taken. This will help to determine what is wrong with your stomach."

4. "This test is carried out in the X-ray Department. You will find it a little uncomfortable, but it's not really painful."

3-26

An adult client is hospitalized with a hiatal hernia. Following a transthoracic hiatal herniorrhaphy, the client returns to the unit with a chest tube attached to a 3-chamber water-seal drainage connected to suction. Which of the following actions should the nurse take initially if the client's chest tube is not draining immediately following surgery?

1. Clamp the chest tube near the point of exit from the chest.

2. Increase the suction applied to the drainage system.

3. Ask the client to deep-breathe and cough.

4. Turn the client toward the operative side.

3-27

The nurse will instruct clients receiving thiaziade drugs to include foods in their diets that are high in:

1. calcium.
2. potassium.
3. iron.
4. magnesium.

3 - 2 8

A client complains of nausea. The nurse administers prochlorperazine maleate 25 mg intramuscularly as prescribed. Following prochlorperazine maleate administration, the nurse will assess the client for:

1 hypotension.
2. headaches.
3. confusion.
4. dry mouth.

3 - 2 9

The nurse is caring for a 3-year-old with chronic liver disease and marked ascites. To promote respiratory function and comfort, the child should be placed in which of the following positions?

1. semi-upright
2. semi-prone
3. dorsal recumbent
4. prone

3 - 3 0

The nurse is giving dietary instructions to mothers of infants and toddlers. The nurse will inform the mothers that diets that include milk to the exclusion of other foods may be deficient in:

1. iron.
2. carbohydrates.
3. vitamin D.
4. vitamin K.

3 - 3 1

A client thought to have cholelithiasis has been hospitalized and scheduled for an ultrasonography. Prior to this diagnostic evaluation, the nurse will:

1. administer a sedative approximately 30 minutes before the procedure.
2. question the client about allergies to iodine and seafood.
3. provide a clear liquid diet the evening before evaluation.
4. provide the client with an explanation of the procedure.

3 - 3 2

As a result of a positive guaiac test on the stools of your client, the physician has prescribed a bland diet. You will provide dietary instruction for the client. Which of the following menus, if selected by the client, would indicate the client is able to identify appropriate meals?

1. hamburger with relish on a roll, ice cream, and coffee
2. ham on rye bread, flavored gelatin, and milk
3. cream cheese on toasted white bread, canned peaches, and decaffeinated coffee
4. bacon, lettuce, and tomato sandwich on whole-wheat bread, applesauce, and tea

3 - 3 3

A 14-year-old is admitted to the hospital for treatment of ulcerative colitis. The client is receiving methantheline bromide. The nurse will explain to the client that the chief purpose of this medication is to:

1. suppress inflammation of the bowel wall.
2. reduce peristaltic activity.
3. neutralize gastrointestinal tract acidity.
4. increase bowel tone.

3 - 3 4

Which groups of food are highest in iron?

1. milk, pork, and squash
2. steak, spinach, and whole-grain bread
3. oranges, chicken, and green beans
4. tomatoes, stawberries, and liver

3 - 3 5

A client was seen in the Emergency Department with severe abdominal pain, nausea, vomiting, and diarrhea. Vital signs were blood pressure 120/80, heart rate 100 beats per minute, respirations 20 breaths per minute, and temperature of 103° F. The client has a history of angina. What was the client's chief complaint?

1. temperature 103°F
2. angina pectoris
3. severe abdominal pain
4. nausea, vomiting, and diarrhea

3 - 3 6

A client receiving antineoplastic agents asks the nurse why the antigout medication allopurinol has been included in the chemotherapy regimen. The nurse's explanation will include the information that allopurinol:

1. enhances the effects of antineoplastic agents.
2. decreases the side effects of nausea and vomiting.
3. will prevent symptoms of gout that may occur due to rapid cell destruction.
4. will prevent destruction of normal cells by promoting folic acid conversion.

3 - 3 7

A client with pancreatitis has an increase in the serum amylase level. This is consistent with a nursing diagnosis of:

1. "altered nutrition, more than body requirements related to excessive intake."
2. "fluid volume excess related to congestive heart failure."
3. "pain related to inflamed pancreas."
4. "altered nutrition, less than body requirements related to inadequate nutrition."

3 - 3 8

A client with a hiatal hernia is receiving the dopamine antagonist metoclopramide hydrochloride. You will explain that the purpose of this medication is to:

1. lower esophageal sphincter pressure.
2. increase gastric emptying.
3. decrease gastric acid production.
4. protect the gastric mucosa.

3 - 3 9

Acid-ash foods for clients with hypercalcemia may be included as part of the treatment of angina. Which of the following will the nurse recognize as foods found on an acid-ash diet?

1. vegetables
2. milk
3. peaches and apples
4. meat

3 - 4 0

Your client has a colostomy. After ambulation, you notice that the client's stoma is a dusky color. You will:

1. have the client lie down and then notify the physician.
2. loosen the drainage pouch and inspect the stoma for ischemia.
3. do nothing since the stoma should appear dusky in color.
4. prepare the client for a stomal irrigation.

3 - 4 1

Which assessment finding is indicative of a vitamin K deficiency?

1. bruising
2. paresthesia
3. brittle nails
4. loss and thinning of hair

3 - 4 2

A 6-month-old infant with phenylketonuria is brought to the clinic. The client is on a phenylalanine-controlled diet. Which information will the nurse include in the teaching plan that emphasizes the cause of this condition?

1. insufficient fat intake during early infancy
2. deficiency of an enzyme needed to utilize galactose during early infancy
3. inability of the infant to metabolize one of the essential amino acids
4. abnormal accumulation of lipids in the cells of infants

3 - 4 3

A client with cirrhosis of the liver is developing hepatic encephalopathy. You will anticipate laboratory studies that will monitor the client's level of:

1. blood ammonia.
2. serum protein.
3. alpha-fetoprotein.
4. serum amylase.

3 - 4 4

A client with cirrhosis of the liver is concerned about spider angiomas on the nose and cheeks. You teach that these are caused by:

1. splenomegaly.
2. decreased prothrombin levels.
3. increased circulating estrogens.
4. urea crystal deposits under the skin.

3 - 4 5

A client has achalasia. To decrease esophageal pressure and improve swallowing, the nurse will anticipate a prescription for:

1. antilipemics.
2. bronchodilators.
3. calcium channel-blockers.
4. anti-infectives.

3 - 4 6

The results of a diagnostic test reveal that a client has salmonellosis. Which of the following measures, if used by the nurse, would be most effective in preventing the transfer of the causative organism of salmonellosis?

1. wearing a protective gown when in proximity to the client
2. discarding any needle used in the treatment of the client
3. washing the hands upon leaving the client's room
4. using disposable dishes for the client's foods

3 - 4 7

After a colonoscopy, which of the following symptoms will suggest that a client has bowel perforation secondary to the procedure?

1. nausea and vomiting
2. abdominal pain and fever
3. abdominal distention and hyperactive bowel sounds
4. hypotension and confusion

3 - 4 8

A client is to have a stool culture for ova and parasites. The accuracy of the results of the client's stool culture would be influenced mostly by which of the following measures taken by the nurse?

1. keeping the specimen warm
2. collecting a large specimen
3. obtaining the specimen before the client has breakfast
4. omitting meat from the client's diet for 3 days

3 - 4 9

A client has liver damage. The nurse will anticipate an abnormally low serum value for:

1. glutaminic-oxaloacitic transaminase.
2. lactic dehydrogenase.
3. albumin.
4. alkaline phosphatase.

3 - 5 0

An adult client is admitted to the hospital with a diagnosis of advanced cirrhosis and ascites. Because the client has advanced cirrhosis of the liver, the nurse would most likely obtain which of the following information during an assessment?

1. clubbing of the fingers
2. an acetone odor of the breath
3. epigastric pain and dysphasia
4. fatigue and muscle wasting

3 - 5 1

A client has been admitted to your unit with a jejunostomy tube. Which nursing action is contraindicated?

1. Administer a bolus tube feeding every 4 hours.
2. Flush the tube with 30 cc of water every 4 hours.
3. Administer medications in liquid form.
4. Change the feeding bag every 24 hours.

3 - 5 2

In planning dietary education for a client on a low-fat diet, the nurse should first:

1. determine a 24-hour recall and a list of foods the client likes best.
2. give the client a list of foods included in a low-fat diet.
3. discuss with the client the important relationship between diet and exercise.
4. tell the client that fruits and vegetables should form the bulk of a low-fat diet.

3 - 5 3

A client is scheduled for a partial glossectomy. The nurse should recognize the primary purpose of oral hygiene pre-operatively is to:

1. reduce the bacterial count in the mouth.
2. alter the pH of the salivary secretions.
3. improve the functioning of the taste buds.
4. promote softening of the lesion.

3 - 5 4

A client receives a diagnosis of acute pancreatitis. In assessing the client's condition, the nurse should expect the laboratory test results to show an elevated serum level of which of the following substances?

1. amylase
2. bilirubin
3. cholesterol
4. gastrin

3 - 5 5

A 6-month-old has been vomiting, crying, and screaming and drawing her knees up to her abdomen for 3 hours. The diagnosis is possible intussusception. Which of the following additional signs of intussusception would the nurse observe and record?

1. jaundice
2. hematuria
3. petechia
4. currant-jellylike stools

3 - 5 6

You are prepared to give potassium chloride liquid to a client with a percutaneous endoscopic gastrostomy who is on continual feedings. Prior to administering the medication, you aspirate 30 cc of residual feed. You will:

1. discard the residual feed and withhold the medication.

2. reinstill the residual feed and give the medication.

3. reinstill the residual feed and hold the medication because potassium chloride may not be given via a percutaneous endoscopic gastrostomy.

4. increase the tube feeding rate and give the medication.

Practice Test 3

Answers, Rationales, and Explanations

3 - 1

③ **The tube feeding container and line are normally changed every 24 hours to prevent transmission of bacteria.**

1. Feedings that have been infusing for more than 8 hours should be discarded. The feeding container and tube, however, do not need to be changed before 24 hours.

2. It is generally not necessary to change the feeding container and the tube before 24 hours.

4. A feeding container and tube are likely to transmit bacteria if not changed after 24 hours of use.

Nursing Process: Evaluating

Client Need: Safe, Effective Care Environment

3 - 2

② **The most accurate assessment for correct placement of a nasogastric tube is an X-ray visualization of the gastric area. With an X ray, one actually sees if the tube is correctly positioned.**

1. Determining the pH of aspirate is one way to check tube placement, but it is not the most accurate way.

3. Auscultation over the gastric area to hear the sound of injected air as it enters the stomach is one method to check the tube placement, but it is not the most accurate.

4. Palpation is not used to determine placement of a nasogastric tube. Injecting enough air to palpate would cause discomfort.

Nursing Process: Implementing

Client Need: Health Promotion and Maintenance

3 - 3

② **The parents should be taught that surgical intervention will not be needed. Medical treatment and allowing time for maturity of the gastrointestinal tract are usually all that is necessary to treat gastroesophageal reflux in the infant. The parents should also be taught to place the infant in an upright position after feedings and during sleep. Medications may be prescribed to hasten emptying the stomach and decrease gastric acidity. If surgery becomes necessary, it is usually beyond infancy. In a technique called fundiplication, the lower esophagus is surrounded by the upper stomach to prevent reflux.**

1. Gastric contents are very acidic and irritating to the respiratory tract if aspirated. The upper sphincter of the stomach is somewhat relaxed in infants and allows for regurgitation of gastric contents. Pneumonia and breathing problems could occur.

3. Formula thickened with rice cereal is a common treatment. The heavier thickened formula is not as likely to reflux and is more likely to empty into the duodenum.

4. Feeding more often and not as much at a time is a common treatment for gastroesophageal reflux. The less full the stomach is, the less likely reflux will occur.

Nursing Process: Evaluating

Client Need: Health Promotion and Maintenance

3 - 4

① **A gastroscopy would probably be the first diagnostic procedure, since upper gastrointestinal bleeding is suspected. A gastroscopy allows direct visualization of the mucosal lining of the esophagus, stomach, and duodenum.**

2. Gastrointestinal X rays would be requested only if the gastroscopy was inconclusive and it was thought that additional information would be useful.

3. Fiberoptic colonoscopy would not be requested since the bleeding is occurring in the upper gastrointestinal tract. A fiberoptic colonoscopy allows direct visualization of the colon up to the ileocecal valve. It is used to diagnose conditions such as inflammatory bowel disease, strictures, and bleeding sites. The procedure also allows for removal of polyps.

4. A gastric analysis is usually requested to analyze the pH and volume of the gastric contents. This test could assist in determining the cause of bleeding, such as high acidity of stomach contents. However, gastric analysis cannot locate specific sites of bleeding since direct visualization is not possible.

Nursing Process: Analyzing

Client Need: Health Promotion and Maintenance

3 - 5

④ **The percutaneous endoscopic gastrostomy (PEG) feeding should be turned off at least 30 minutes prior to the weighing process. This will decrease the risk of aspiration.**

1. Weighing the day's feeding formula and adding it to the client's weight is not an appropriate or common practice.
2. Clients receiving continuous PEG feedings can be weighed on bed scales.
3. There is no clinical reason to defer the daily weighings.

Nursing Process: Implementing
Client Need: Safe, Effective Care Environment

3 - 6

② **You will instruct clients to hold the abdomen firmly, take several deep breaths, and then cough 2 or 3 times as they exhale. Effective splinting of the surgical site will allow the client to breathe deeply and cough more effectively. The client will experience less pain since stress on the suture line is relieved. The goal of coughing and deep breathing is to fully expand and aerate the lungs, thus allowing secretions to be coughed out. Effective coughing is always preceded by deep breathing.**

1. When possible, the nurse should teach the postoperative client to maintain a sitting (upright) position for coughing and deep breathing exercises. This position lowers abdominal organs and allows the diaphragm to expand fully. However, a sitting position may not be therapeutic for all surgical clients.
3. The client should not tighten the stomach muscles when coughing and deep breathing exercises are performed. Also, it is not necessary that coughing should be forceful. It would be helpful to have the client slightly flex the knees to take tension off the abdomen.
4. The client should be taught to breathe deeply from the diaphragm. Raising the shoulders tends to facilitate shallow breathing, not deep breathing.

Nursing Process: Implementing
Client Need: Physiological Integrity

3 - 7

④ Ingestion of caffeine and chocolate may exacerbate gastroesophageal reflux. The reflux of stomach contents into the esophagus is due in part to a lowering of esophageal sphincter pressure. Certain foods have been found to lower the sphincter's pressure. These foods include caffeine, chocolate, peppermint, and fatty foods.

1, 2, and 3. Neither poultry, pastas, herbs, or spices have been found to significantly lower esophageal sphincter pressure.

Nursing Process: Assessing
Client Need: Health Promotion and Maintenance

3 - 8

④ Administering potassium chloride will replace the potassium that is being lost through vomiting. Potassium is one of the electrolytes contained in gastric secretions. When excessive vomiting or suctioning of gastric contents occurs, clients lose potassium (K+). If potassium is not replaced, hypokalemia may occur.

1. Potassium is usually lost in urine output during diuretic therapy.
2. Potassium cannot be stored in the body. A 40 mEq of potassium must be consumed daily. A normal potassium level is 3.5 to 5.5 mEq/L.
3. Potassium does not promote excretion of sodium. When potassium is lost from cells, sodium shifts into the cells to replace lost K+.

Nursing Process: Evaluating
Client Need: Physiological Integrity

3 - 9

① The dumping syndrome is a direct result of removing a large portion of the stomach. The dumping syndrome is a set of unpleasant vasomotor and gastrointestinal (GI) symptoms that occur after consuming a meal in 10 to 50% of clients who have had gastric surgery. Food passes too rapidly from the stomach remnant. Symptoms include weakness, faintness, cramping, and diarrhea.

2. Hyperosmolar chyme occurs as a result of food entering the jejunum without proper mixing.

3 and 4. The dumping syndrome occurs as a direct result of gastrointestinal surgery. Eating large quantities of food, not lying down after meals, and drinking liquids with the meal contributes to the problem.

Nursing Process: Implementing
Client Need: Physiological Integrity

3 - 1 0

③ **Most commercially prepared formulas contains about 20 kcal/oz, as does breast milk. Some of the formulas made for preterm infants are slightly higher in energy. The following equation may be used to calculate the ounces of formula for a given energy:**

$$\frac{1 \text{ oz}}{20 \text{ kcal}} \times 500 \text{ kcal} = 25 \text{ oz}.$$

1. 5 oz of formula would contain only 100 kcal of energy.

2 and 4. 15 oz and 50 oz of formula would contain 300 and 1000 kcal of energy respectively.

Nursing Process: Assessing
Client Need: Health Promotion and Maintenance

3 - 1 1

② **Babies require 105 to 110 kcal/kg/day of energy. The following formula may be used to calculate this infant's caloric needs:**

$$\frac{105 \text{ to } 110 \text{ kcal/kg}}{\text{day}} \times \frac{1 \text{ kg}}{2.2 \text{ lb}} \times 10 \text{ lbs} = \frac{477 \text{ to } 500 \text{ kcal}}{\text{day}}.$$

1, 3, and 4. A baby requiring 500 kcal/day would be undernourished receiving only 100 kcal/day, and overfed receiving either 1,000 or 1,500 kcal/day.

Nursing Process: Assessing
Client Need: Health Promotion and Maintenance

3 - 1 2

① **Manifestations of Crohn's disease include diarrhea, fatigue, abdominal pain, and weight loss. Crohn's disease is a chronic, nonspecific inflammatory disorder of unknown origin that can affect any part of the gastrointestinal (GI) tract. It is characterized by inflammation of segments of the GI tract. This condition is also called regional ileitis and regional enteritis.**

2. Jaundice and steatorrhea (fatty stools) are symptoms of gallbladder disease.

3. Shortness of breath and tachycardia would be symptoms manifested in a client with chronic obstructive pulmonary disease (COPD).

4. Dependent edema and ascites are seen in right-sided congestive heart failure.

Nursing Process: Analyzing
Client Need: Physiological Integrity

3 - 1 3

③ **Prolonged gastrosophageal disease can quickly become life threatening, causing esophageal ulceration. A repeated assault on the esophageal mucosa by acid reflux can cause erosion of the esophagus and hemorrhage. This is an uncommon occurrence, but can be morbid if not treated promptly. Symptoms often become very severe and constant with little relief from previously effective treatments. This is a medical emergency.**

1 and 2. Neither pharyngitis nor colitis are directly related to gastroesophageal reflux disease (GERD). However, they may occur simultaneously.

4. The chest pains associated with angina may easily be confused with the "heartburn" associated with GERD, and vice versa. Although one does not necessarily cause the other, pain that may be cardiac in origin must always be considered when a client complains of chest pain.

Nursing Process: Analyzing
Client Need: Physiological Integrity

3 - 1 4

② **Baked chicken breast, apple, and skim milk would be appropriate foods for a client with hypercholesterolemia. Clients with hypercholesterolemia have elevated serum cholesterol levels, which have been found to contribute to the development of coronary artery disease. The consumption of low-fat foods, such as white meats, fruits, vegetables, grains, and skimmed or nonfat dairy products will help lower serum lipid levels.**

1, 3, and 4. Beef, cheese, fried foods, and processed meats are all high in fat and contribute to hypercholesterolemia.

Nursing Process: Evaluating
Client Need: Health Promotion and Maintenance

3 - 1 5

④ **You will suspect a pharyngoesophageal diverticulum. A diverticulum is an outpouching of the mucosa that protrudes through a weak place in the esophageal musculature. Symptoms include dysphagia, belching, regurgitation of undigested food, gurgling sounds after eating (caused by fluid and food filling the diverticulum), coughing caused by tracheal irritation, halitosis (bad breath), and a sour taste in the mouth caused by decomposing food lodged in the diverticulum.**

1. A diffuse esophageal spasm is due to motor excitement of the esophagus that produces alternate periods of contractions and relaxation. Symptoms include dysphagia (difficulty swallowing) and chest pain.

2. Gastroesophageal reflux is characterized by reflux (backward flow) of the acidic contents of the stomach into the distal portion of the esophagus. Symptoms include pyrosis (heartburn), regurgitation (return of food from the stomach into the esophagus and mouth), dysphagia (difficulty swallowing), and a painful feeling of a lump in the throat.

3. Hiatal hernia Type 1 is a sliding hernia where the upper stomach and the gastroesophageal junction are pushed upward in and out of the thorax. Type 2 is a herniation of a portion of the stomach through an opening (hiatus) into the esophagus. This condition is also known as esophageal or diaphragmatic hernia. Symptoms of Types 1 and 2 include pyrosis (heartburn) and dysphagia (difficulty swallowing).

Nursing Process: Assessing
Client Need: Physiological Integrity

3 - 1 6

③ **Pyloric obstruction is suspected. Scarring at the pylorus is likely to cause pyloric obstruction. As a result of the obstruction, the contents of the stomach are unable to empty properly, which causes gastric fullness, distention, pain, nausea, and vomiting. When clients lie down at night, pain intensifies since the stomach is even less likely to be emptied by peristalsis.**

1. The symptoms of peptic ulcer perforation are different from those of pyloric obstruction. Symptoms of peptic ulcer perforation include sudden onset of severe upper abdominal pain that spreads rapidly throughout the abdomen as the gastrointestinal contents spill into the peritoneal cavity. Clients experience a rigid boardlike abdomen. Respirations become shallow and rapid, and bacterial septicemia develops, causing fever and hypovolemic shock.

2. Some of the symptoms of acute gastritis are similar to those of pyloric obstruction. However, the client's history of scarring at the distal end of the pyloric sphincter is highly suggestive of pyloric obstruction.

4. A paralytic ileus is a postoperative complication. Peristalsis in a portion of the bowel stops, which causes diminished or absent bowel sounds. Abdominal distention occurs and the client complains of pain and feelings of fullness. A nasogastric tube is usually required to relieve distention and vomiting until normal bowel peristalsis resumes.

Nursing Process: Assessing
Client Need: Physiological Integrity

3 - 1 7

(4) **The nurse should explain to the client that 90 to 100% of clients experiencing ulcerative colitis have blood, pus, and mucus in their stools. Understanding the nature and symptoms of the disease process may help to alleviate the client's anxiety.**

1. It is not necessary to check the client's stools for the presence of occult blood since blood in the stools is a typical finding. 90 to 100% of clients in the acute phase of ulcerative colitis have blood in their stools.

2. The client should participate in maintaining a record of the number and description of stools. However, simply maintaining a record will not give the client the information needed to allay anxiety about blood in the stools.

3. It is not necessary to notify the client's physician since blood in the stools is expected in ulcerative colitis. Nursing care would include a record of the number and description of stools.

Nursing Process: Implementing
Client Need: Psychosocial Integrity

3 - 1 8

(1) **The normal serum bilirubin level is 0.2 to 1.0 mg/dL. A serum bilirubin level of 50 mg/dL is associated with late-stage liver disease.**

2, 3, and 4. Serum bilirubin levels higher than 1.0 mg/dL are outside the normal range.

Nursing Process: Evaluating
Client Need: Physiological Integrity

3 - 1 9

(2) **The colostomy should begin to function in 2 to 4 days. It generally takes this long for peristalsis to be restored following abdominal surgery.**

1. It is not usual for a colostomy to function as soon as 12 to 24 hours since peristalsis doesn't return for 48 to 72 hours postoperatively.

3 and 4. A colostomy should begin to function in response to the return of peristalsis. Peristalsis should return between 2 to 4 days postoperatively. If peristalsis has not returned, complications such as a paralytic ileus may be suspected.

Nursing Process: Implementing
Client Need: Psychosocial Integrity

3-20

③ **Offering frequent small portions of favorite foods following periods of rest will prevent exhaustion in the acutely ill child and will meet nutritional requirements.**

1. The temperature of the food is not the issue. The foods should require little energy to consume and should be enjoyed by the child.
2. Providing liquids through a straw would conserve energy. However, if the child does not like the liquids, they are not likely to be consumed.
4. If there are no foods that the child enjoys in the regularly scheduled meals, they are not likely to be consumed.

Nursing Process: Implementing
Client Need: Health Promotion and Maintenance

3-21

④ **The sump drain will allow wound healing to take place from its lowest depth without forming an abscess.**

1. The character and volume of drainage can be assessed by using a sump drain. However, this is not the primary purpose for the drain.
2. Flatus will be expelled from the colostomy, not the perineal wound.
3. A sump drain can be as easily contaminated as a dressing.

Nursing Process: Evaluating
Client Need: Physiological Integrity

3-22

④ **Aluminum hydroxide (Amphojel) is an antacid that neutralizes gastric secretions by buffering hydrochloric acid.**

1. Antiulcer (histamine H2) antagonists such as Tagamet inhibit the secretion of hydrochloride acid, not antacids like Amphojel.
2 and 3. Aluminum hydroxide does not affect the breakdown of protein or absorb air that has been swallowed.

Nursing Process: Implementing
Client Need: Physiological Integrity

3-23

② The purpose of the infusion is to replace the potassium that is lost through vomiting. Potassium is one of the electrolytes contained in gastric secretions. Excessive vomiting or suctioning of gastric contents results in potassium loss and, if not replaced, can lead to hypokalemia.

1. There is no indication that potassium is being lost through urinary output. Clients who are treated with diuretics such as furosemide (Lasix) may lose potassium. However, there is no indication that this client is receiving a diuretic.

3. Dietary sources of potassium are not stored in the body. People of all ages need to consume potassium on a daily basis. Foods high in potassium include dried peach halves, lima beans, winter squash, potatoes, bananas, and pinto beans.

4. Potassium does not promote excretion of sodium chloride.

Nursing Process: Implementing
Client Need: Physiological Integrity

3-24

② A combination of 30 grams of powdered skim milk and 1 whole egg will provide the highest amount of protein.

1, 3, and 4. Light cream, corn syrup, ice cream, chocolate syrup, and sugar are high in fat and sugar and would not be encouraged.

Nursing Process: Planning
Client Need: Health Promotion and Maintenance

3-25

① An explanation by the nurse that is accurate and appropriate would be, "In the X-ray Department, you will be asked to drink a thick liquid, and then several X rays of the upper part of your digestive tract will be taken at intervals." This explanation is simple, factual, and understandable to a lay person or a client.

2. A gastrointestinal series (GI series) does not require the client to swallow a tube.

3. The substance used for performing a GI series is radiopaque, not radioactive.

4. A GI series is not uncomfortable.

Nursing Process: Implementing
Client Need: Safe, Effective Care Environment

3-26

③ If a client's chest tube is not draining immediately following a transthoracic hiatal herniorrhaphy, the nurse should have the client deep-breathe and cough. In the immediate postoperative period, bloody drainage is expected. Having the client deep-breathe and cough will effect changes in intrapleural pressures and, by observing for oscillation of the fluid in the water-seal chamber of the drainage apparatus, it will be possible to determine if the chest tube and connecting tubing are patent. If plugged, the increased intrapleural pressure manifested during coughing may be sufficient to dislodge any obstruction. A patent system is necessary to prevent a hemo- or pneumothorax.

1. Clamping the chest tube may be done when checking for an air leak. However, clamping of chest tubes is not done when the chest tubes are not draining.

2. Increasing the suction will draw in air through the vented tubing. It will not affect drainage.

4. The client should be turned toward the operative site after coughing and deep breathing.

Nursing Process: Implementing
Client Need: Safe, Effective Care Environment

3-27

② The nurse should instruct clients on thiazide drugs such as chlorothiazide (Diuril) to include foods in their diet that are high in potassium. Thiazide diuretics are potassium depleting. Foods high in potassium include peaches, lima beans, winter squash, pears, baked potatoes with skin, bananas, and oranges.

1, 3, and 4. Calcium, iron, and magnesium are not affected by thiazide diuretics.

Nursing Process: Implementing
Client Need: Physiological Integrity

3-28

① The nurse should assess the client for hypotension following prochlorperazine maleate (Compazine) administration. Hypotension is an adverse reaction to prochlorperazine maleate. Other side effects include drowsiness, dizziness, contact dermatitis, and photosensitivity.

2, 3, and 4. Headache, confusion, and dry mouth are not associated with Compazine administration.

Nursing Process: Assessing
Client Need: Safe, Effective Care Environment

3-29

(1) **The child should be placed in a semi-upright (45-degree) position. A semi-upright position affords maximum lung expansion for the client with ascites. The recumbent position restricts diaphragmatic excursion.**

2. The semi-prone position (client lying on abdomen with head of bed slightly elevated) would not facilitate breathing.

3. A dorsal recumbent position (client lying on back) would not facilitate breathing.

4. A prone position (client lying on abdomen face down) would be very uncomfortable and would obstruct breathing by pressing the fluid in the abdomen (ascites) up against the diaphragm.

Nursing Process: Implementing
Client Need: Physiological Integrity

3-30

(1) **The nurse will inform the mothers that diets that include milk to the exclusion of other foods may be deficient in iron. Infants and children between the ages of 6 and 34 months may be vulnerable to iron-deficiency anemia since cow's milk is low in iron. Breast-fed infants or those receiving iron-fortified formula usually receive adequate iron intake.**

2, 3, and 4. Cow's milk is not deficient in carbohydrates or vitamins D and K.

Nursing Process: Implementing
Client Need: Health Promotion and Maintenance

3-31

(4) **The nurse will provide the client with an explanation of the ultrasonography and its purpose.**

1. A sedative is not necessary for clients having ultrasonography. There is no pain or discomfort as the transducer glides over the surface of the body.

2. Ultrasonography does not require the client to ingest a contrast media that might cause an allergic reaction.

3. Special dietary preparation is not needed for ultrasonography. However, the client should be instructed not to eat solid food 12 hours before the procedure. The client may have water.

Nursing Process: Implementing
Client Need: Psychological Integrity

3 - 3 2

③ **Cream cheese on toasted white bread, canned peaches, and decaffeinated coffee are foods that are allowed on a bland diet.**

1, 2, and 4. Foods that are not allowed on a bland diet include fried foods, cured meats, high-fiber breads, highly seasoned foods, and food or drinks that contain caffeine.

Nursing Process: Evaluating
Client Need: Health Promotion and Maintenance

3 - 3 3

② **The nurse will inform the client that gastrointestinal peristaltic activity will be reduced. Methantheline bromide (Banthine) has an anticholinergic action that inhibits motility in the gastrointestinal tract. This medication is used as an antispasmodic in the treatment of clients with hypermotility of the intestine and colon.**

1. Banthine does not affect inflammation. Sulfonamides such as sulfasalazine (Azulifidine) or sulfisoxazole (Gantrisin) are often administered for their anti-inflammatory effects.

3. An antacid such as Amphojel, milk of magnesia, or Maalox would neutralize gastrointestinal tract acidity.

4. Banthine does not affect bowel tone.

Nursing Process: Implementing
Client Need: Physiological Integrity

3 - 3 4

② **Steak, spinach, and whole-grain breads are high in iron. Other foods high in iron include muscle meats, eggs, dried fruits, legumes, dark green leafy vegetables, potatoes, enriched bread, and cereals.**

1, 3, and 4. Milk, pork, squash, oranges, chicken, green beans, tomatoes, strawberries, and liver are not high in iron.

Nursing Process: Implementing
Client Need: Physiological Integrity

3 - 3 5

③ **Severe abdominal pain was the client's chief complaint. The severe abdominal pain is what brought the client to the hospital.**

1. The client's temperature is part of the present health status.
2. Angina pectoris is a part of the client's past history.
4. Nausea, vomiting, and diarrhea are a part of the history of the present illness.

Nursing Process: Assessing
Client Need: Physiological Integrity

3 - 3 6

③ **Allopurinol (Zyloprim) prevents the symptoms of gout that may occur due to rapid cell destruction caused by antineoplastic medications.**

1. Zyloprim does not enhance the effects of antineoplastic agents.
2. Zyloprim is not an antiemetic and will not decrease nausea and vomiting.
4. Zyloprim does not prevent destruction of normal cells.

Nursing Process: Implementing
Client Need: Psychological Integrity

3 - 3 7

③ **A client with pancreatitis who has an increase in serum amylase level will have a nursing diagnosis of "pain related to inflamed pancreas." An elevation in serum amylase and lipase is consistent with pancreatitis. A common clinical manifestation of pancreatitis is pain.**

1. An increase in the serum cholesterol level may be seen with an increase in food intake.
2. A decrease in the serum sodium level may suggest the increased fluid volume seen with congestive heart failure.
4. Hypoalbuminemia is seen with inadequate intake of nutrients.

Nursing Process: Analyzing
Client Need: Physiological Integrity

3-38

② **Metoclopramide (Reglan) increases the resting tone of the lower esophageal sphincter and facilitates gastric emptying. Persons with hiatal hernia usually receive the dopamine antagonist metoclopramide (Reglan). This medication stimulates motility of the upper gastrointestinal tract without stimulating gastric secretions.**

1. Reglan does not lower esophageal sphincter pressure.
3. Reglan is an antiemetic, gastrointestinal stimulant. It does not decrease gastric acid production.
4. Medications such as Sulcralfate protect the gastric mucosa, not Reglan.

Nursing Process: Implementing
Client Need: Physiological Integrity

3-39

④ **Acid-ash foods include protein-rich choices such as meat, fish, poultry, eggs, cheese, grains (breads and cereals), and certain fruits (cranberries, prunes, and plums).**

1 and 3. Vegetables and most fruits are not rich in protein and are therefore not included in an acid-ash diet.
2. Milk is high in calcium and would not be recommended for clients who are experiencing hypercalcemia.

Nursing Process: Planning
Client Need: Health Promotion and Maintenance

3-40

② **The drainage pouch should be loosened and the stoma inspected for ischemia. A dusky color indicates stomal ischemia. Blood supply may be promoted by loosening or adjusting the colostomy pouch. If this does not correct the deficiency of blood supply, the physician should be notified.**

1. The nurse would examine the client's stoma to determine the possible cause for the ischemia before notifying the physician.
3. A healthy stoma is pink.
4. Irrigating the colostomy would not affect the color of the stoma.

Nursing Process: Implementing
Client Need: Physiological Integrity

3 - 4 1

(1) **When there is a deficiency in vitamin K, the client's blood will not clot easily, and therefore bruising would be evident. Vitamin K plays an important role in blood coagulation.**

2. Paresthesia is indicative of vitamin B12 deficiencies, not vitamin K deficiencies.

3 and 4. Brittle nails, hair thinning, and hair loss are consistent with protein deficiency, not vitamin K.

Nursing Process: Analyzing
Client Need: Physiological Integrity

3 - 4 2

(3) **In phenylketonuria (PKU), the hepatic enzyme needed to metabolize the amino acid phenylalanine (an essential amino acid formed from protein) is absent, resulting in the accumulation of phenylalanine in the bloodstream and excretion of phenyl acid in the urine.**

1. Phenylketonuria is not associated with fat intake.

2. Galactose is a monosaccharide, not an amino acid. Galactose is readily absorbed in the digestive tract and is converted into glycogen in the liver.

4. "Lipids" is a descriptive term rather than a chemical name such as protein and carbohydrate. Lipids do not affect the essential amino acid phenylalanine.

Nursing Process: Implementing
Client Need: Health Promotion and Maintenance

3 - 4 3

(1) **The blood ammonia level will be elevated in clients with hepatic encephalopathy (hepatic coma). The conversion of ammonia to urea normally occurs in the liver; therefore, the ammonia level will be elevated when the liver is affected with cirrhosis.**

2. Serum protein refers to any of several proteins in the blood serum. Serum protein levels above or below the normal range do not directly affect the conversion of ammonia to urea.

3. Alpha-fetoprotein refers to an antigen present in the human fetus. Elevated levels of alpha-fetoprotein are also found in adults with hepatic carcinomas or chemical injuries. Alpha-fetoprotein does not directly affect the conversion of ammonia to urea.

4. Serum amylase is a class of enzyme that splits up starches. When the enzyme is found in animals, the enzyme is referred to as A-amylase. When found in plants, the enzyme is referred to as B-amylase. Serum amylase does not directly affect the conversion of ammonia to urea.

Nursing Process: Analyzing
Client Need: Physiological Integrity

3 - 4 4

③ Spider angiomas are caused by an increase in circulating estrogen as a result of the liver's inability to inactivate it. Spider angiomas are small dilated blood vessels with a bright red center and spidery branches. They appear on the nose, cheeks, upper trunk, neck, and shoulders of clients with cirrhosis of the liver.

1. Splenomegaly refers to enlargement of the spleen and does not cause spider angiomas. However, splenomegaly may be present in cirrhosis of the liver.

2. Prothrombin is a chemical substance in the circulating blood. Prothrombin is produced by thrombokinase interacting with calcium salts. Prothrombin is not directly associated with spider angiomas.

4. Urea crystals on the skin is associated with renal failure. However, due to aggressive and early treatments, it is uncommon today.

Nursing Process: Implementing
Client Need: Physiological Integrity

3 - 4 5

③ The nurse will anticipate a prescription for calcium channel-blockers. Achalasia is the absence of, or ineffective, peristalsis in the distal portion of the esophagus. It is associated with failure of the esophageal sphincter to relax and permit swallowing. Calcium channel-blockers reduce esophageal pressure and thereby improve swallowing by reducing arterial resistance.

1. Antilipemics are agents that prevent or counteract the buildup of fatty substances in the blood. Antilipemics do not affect esophageal pressure.

2. Bronchodilators dilate the bronchus. They do not affect esophageal pressure.

4. Anti-infectives do not affect esophageal pressure. However, they may be administered for the treatment of aspiration pneumonia that can occur with esophageal spillover.

Nursing Process: Planning
Client Need: Physiological Integrity

3 - 4 6

③ The nursing measure that would be most effective in preventing the transfer of the salmonella organism is handwashing.

1. Gown and gloves must be worn by individuals when in direct contact with infected clients.

2. The use of proper handwashing technique by all individuals entering and leaving the room will be most effective in preventing the spread of infection.

4. Using disposable dishes for the client's food is also effective in preventing the spread of infection of salmonella. However, handwashing is the most effective measure in preventing the transfer of salmonella.

Nursing Process: Implementing
Client Need: Safe, Effective Care Environment

3 - 4 7

② **Following a colonoscopy, abdominal pain and fever directly suggest bowel perforation and occurrence of peritonitis secondary to perforation.**

1, 3, and 4. Indirect suggestions of perforation include distension, hyperactive bowel sounds, hypotension, confusion, nausea, and vomiting.

Nursing Process: Assessing
Client Need: Physiological Integrity

3 - 4 8

① **The accuracy of the result of a stool specimen for ova and parasites is dependent upon the specimen being fresh and warm. Ova and parasites will not live in temperatures much lower than the normal body temperature. Contamination with urine will destroy parasites in a specimen.**

2. Collecting a large specimen is not necessary. A small amount of feces will provide results for ova and parasites.

3. Obtaining the specimen before the client has breakfast is not necessary. However, the specimen does need to be fresh and warm.

4. Omitting meat from the client's diet for 3 days has no impact on a specimen for ova and parasites.

Nursing Process: Implementing
Client Need: Safe, Effective Care Environment

3 - 4 9

③ **The nurse would expect a client with liver damage to have abnormally low serum values of albumin. Liver damage is characterized by decreased ability of the liver to synthesize proteins. Consequently, albumin synthesis is reduced.**

1. Serum glutaminic-oxaloacitic transaminase (SGOT) is an enzyme present in serum and body tissue. An elevation of SGOT is associated with myocardial infarction or hepatic cell damage.

2. Lactic dehydrogenase (LDH) is an enzyme found in various tissues and serum. LDH is important in catalyzing the oxidation of lactate. It has a direct impact on liver damage.

4. Alkaline phosphatase (ALP) is an enzyme originating mainly in the bone, liver, and placenta and with some activity in the kidney and intestine. It has a direct affect in clients with liver damage.

Nursing Process: Assessing
Client Need: Physiological Integrity

3 - 5 0

④ **When assessing a client with advanced cirrhosis and ascites, the nurse would observe muscle wasting and signs of fatigue. Chronic cirrhosis and malnutrition affect carbohydrate and protein metabolism, leading to generalized weakness, fatigue, and muscle wasting.**

1. Clubbing of the fingers is an indication of a heart condition due to ischemia.
2. An acetone odor of breath could indicate diabetic ketoacidosis.
3. Epigastric pain and dysphagia could indicate a gastrointestinal problem.

Nursing Process: Assessing
Client Need: Physiological Integrity

3 - 5 1

① **Because a jejunostomy tube introduces food directly into the jejunum, a bolus feeding is contraindicated. A bolus feeding would cause a hyperosmolar reaction much like the dumping syndrome. Clients with a jejunostomy tube will need continuous enteral feeding.**

2. The nurse will need to flush the tube with 30 cc of water every 4 hours.
3. The nurse will need to administer medications in a liquid form.
4. The nurse will need to change the feeding bag every 24 hours.

Nursing Process: Planning
Client Need: Safe, Effective Care Environment

3 - 5 2

① **The nurse should first determine a 24-hour recall and a list of foods the client likes best. The client's eating habits and lifestyle should also be considered. This will help the nurse plan an acceptable diet, thus increasing chances of compliance.**

2, 3, and 4. Providing lists of food, education, and telling the client about fruits and vegetables is less helpful. The nurse should first complete 24-hour recall of the foods the client likes.

Nursing Process: Planning
Client Need: Health Promotion and Maintenance

3 - 5 3

① The primary purpose of preoperative oral hygiene in clients scheduled for a partial glossectomy is to reduce the bacterial count in the mouth. Measures to increase the cleanliness of the oral cavity before surgery will reduce the incidence of postoperative infections such as surgical parotitis.

2. Preoperative oral hygiene is not given to alter the pH of salivary secretions.

3. Preoperative oral hygiene is not given to improve the function of the taste buds.

4. Preoperative oral hygiene is not given to soften lesions.

Nursing Process: Analyzing

Client Need: Physiological Integrity

3 - 5 4

① A client with acute pancreatitis will show an elevated serum amylase. Serum amylase levels increase due to activation of this enzyme while it is still in the pancreas. This causes actual tissue damage and autodigestion of the pancreas.

2. Bilirubin is produced from the hemoglobin of red blood cells. It is changed chemically in the liver and excreted in the bile. The accumulation of bilirubin leads to jaundice. Bilirubin does not directly affect the pancreas or cause pancreatitis.

3. Cholesterol is a component in cell membrane and plasma lipoproteins. It is absorbed from the diet and synthesized in the liver and other body tissues. Elevated cholesterol may indicate a risk for pancreatitis and other disorders. However, in acute pancreatitis, there will be a marked increase in amylase.

4. Gastrin refers to a group of hormones secreted by the mucosa of the pyloric area of the stomach. Gastrin affects the secretionary activity of the gallbladder, pancreas, and small intestine. However, it does not directly cause an increase in amylase.

Nursing Process: Assessing

Client Need: Physiological Integrity

3 - 5 5

④ The nurse will observe and record currant-jellylike stools. Currant-jellylike stools are caused by blood and mucus in the intestinal tract. Other symptoms are absence of stools, increasing abdominal distention and tenderness, sausage-like mass in the upper right abdomen, dehydration, fever, and a shocklike state.

1, 2, and 3. Jaundice, hematuria, and petechia are not signs commonly associated with intussusception.

Nursing Process: Analyzing

Client Need: Physiological Integrity

3 - 5 6

② **You will reinstill the residual feed into the percutaneous endoscopic gastrostomy (PEG) and give the medication. Reinstillation of the residual volume helps avoid fluid and electrolyte imbalance.**

1. Residual volumes are usually reinstilled. There is no reason to withhold the medication.
3. Potassium chloride liquid may be given via the PEG.
4. There is no indication that the tube feeding rate should be increased.

Nursing Process: Implementing
Client Need: Physiological Integrity

Practice Test 4

Immune and Lymphatic/Hematological Systems and Cancer

4 - 1

A client's wound has eviscerated. Which of the following will you implement?

1. Stay with the client and notify the physician.
2. Apply a clean, dry dressing to the wound.
3. Cleanse the wound with Betadine and apply bacteriostatic ointment.
4. Place sterile towels soaked in sterile saline over the wound.

4 - 2

A child who is due for an immunization should not receive that immunization if the child:

1. has recently been exposed to an infectious disease.
2. is receiving antimicrobial (antibiotic) therapy.
3. has a moderately severe illness, without fever.
4. had a moderate local reaction to a previous vaccine injection.

4 - 3

An early symptom of hepatitis A is:

1. loss of appetite.
2. abdominal distention.
3. ecchymosis.
4. shortness of breath.

4 - 4

Which of the following statements is true regarding chemotherapy-related alopecia?

1. Hair loss is temporary; growth will occur soon after chemotherapy is discontinued.
2. Hair loss is transient and is one of the minor side effects of chemotherapy.
3. Hair loss can be minimized by adjusting the dosage of the causative medication.
4. Hair loss is permanent so clients need to prepare for alternatives such as wigs.

4 - 5

An infant has hemolytic disease of the newborn. The nurse caring for the infant should teach the parents that the development of jaundice in the newborn is caused by:

1. polycythemia.
2. an abnormal production of melanin.
3. excessive destruction of red blood cells.
4. hypobilirubinemia.

4 - 6

Following a lumpectomy for breast cancer, the cyclophosphamide, methotrexate, fluorouracil protocol was prescribed. Which of the following statements should be included in the teaching plan of the client receiving these medications?

1. Have the client see a cardiologist prior to chemotherapy.
2. Encourage the client to increase fluid intake to approximately 3 liters per day.
3. See that the client protects herself from sun during chemotherapy.
4. Recommend that the client eat only foods she likes because of potential nausea.

4 - 7

A 60-year-old has terminal lung cancer. On admission, a morphine drip was prescribed to treat intractable pain. Which of the following would the nurse recognize as a side effect of this medication?

1. Client is awake and alert and requires minimal rescue doses of medication for pain.
2. Client requires rescue doses of pain medication every 4 hours.
3. Client has not had a bowel movement for 5 days.
4. Client's pulse rate is 60 beats per minute.

4 - 8

A 3-year-old with hemophilia (factor VIII deficiency) was admitted to the hospital because of persistent bleeding from a minor laceration. In planning care, the nurse will anticipate which of the following consequences of hospitalization to be most traumatic for the client?

1. inhibition from running about freely
2. separation from family
3. placement in an unfamiliar environment
4. disruption of routines and rituals

4 - 9

A client is admitted to the medical-surgical unit with a diagnosis of anemia. The laboratory results reveal a hemoglobin of 6.8 gm/dL. Which therapy do you anticipate?

1. No therapy is anticipated; this is a normal hemoglobin count.
2. albumin intravenously
3. 1 unit of packed red blood cells
4. normal saline intravenously

4 - 1 0

A 41-year-old is admitted to the hospital with chronic granulocytic leukemia. The client also has anemia and thrombocytopenia. Because the client has thrombocytopenia, the nurse should include which of the following measures in the client's plan of care?

1. placing the client in a semi-upright position
2. limiting the client's intake of fluids
3. protecting the client from injury
4. exercising the client's lower extremities

4 - 1 1

Which of the following measures should the nurse implement to control bleeding into the joints of a client who is experiencing hemarthrosis?

1. Begin gentle passive exercises.
2. Immobilize the joint in an elastic compression bandage to apply pressure.
3. Wrap the joint in an elastic compression bandage to prevent bleeding.
4. Apply a tourniquet above the joint.

4 - 1 2

A client who is receiving chemotherapy for treatment of breast cancer tells you that she notices her mouth is extremely dry all the time. You know this is probably a side effect of chemotherapy, and is called:

1. xerostomia.
2. alopecia.
3. xanthoma.
4. anemia.

4 - 1 3

A client has sickle-cell anemia. The nurse's assessment of the client is least likely to reveal:

1. paleness of hands and soles of feet.
2. height and weight retardation.
3. elevated heart rate with no cyanosis.
4. several fresh bruises on the calves of the legs.

4 - 1 4

A client is to receive a blood transfusion. Prior to administration of the blood, it is important for the nurse to:

1. instruct the client that the transfusion takes less than 30 minutes.
2. administer an antibiotic.
3. infuse dextrose 5% in water with the blood.
4. verify the prescription and check labels carefully with another nurse.

4 - 1 5

An 8-year-old has rubella. Which of the following recommendations will the nurse stress regarding contact with others?

1. "Do not let the child play with brothers and sisters until there is no longer a rash."
2. "Do not allow friends or relatives who are pregnant to visit for at least 5 days after the rash disappears."
3. "Do not allow your children to sleep with each other until a week after the rash disappears."
4. "Do not allow your children to play with other children in the neighborhood for several days."

4 - 1 6

A client who has been receiving chemotherapy for liver cancer is making holiday plans. The client's white blood cell count today is 2000/cm³. Which of the following is the most appropriate advice to give this client regarding holiday plans?

1. "You should avoid being with your family because you may be contagious."
2. "There is little point in celebrating this year, isn't there?"
3. "Try not to eat foods that are high in carbohydrates over the holidays."
4. "You should try to avoid being in crowded public situations."

4 - 1 7

Which of the following immunizations should not be given to a 2-month-old infant whose caregiver is currently receiving chemotherapy?

1. oral polio vaccine
2. hepatitis B
3. diphtheria, tetanus, and pertussis
4. Haemophilus type B

4 - 1 8

A client who has leukemia has a platelet count of 50 cells x 109/L. Nursing care must include which of the following?

1. scheduled analgesia, since a low platelet count is associated with profound muscle pain
2. measures to prevent bleeding and bruising
3. parenteral medications only, since GI absorption will be poor
4. vigorous range-of-motion exercises

4 - 1 9

A young child will receive the Haemophilus influenzae type B vaccine. The nurse will teach the child's parents that the vaccine will:

1. protect the child from one cause of serious infections such as epiglottitis or meningitis.
2. protect the child from hepatitis B disease.
3. help prevent human immunodeficiency virus disease in young children.
4. help prevent influenza.

4-20

Clients experiencing acute hepatitis B should be advised to avoid:

1. citrus juices.
2. sleeping on their right sides.
3. antihistamines for their pruritus.
4. contact sports.

4-21

A client who has been diagnosed with autoimmune chronic hepatitis will have which of the following laboratory results?

1. a positive hepatitis B surface antigen
2. low liver function tests
3. elevated liver function tests
4. low serum bilirubin levels

4-22

Which of the following laboratory studies indicates an infectious process?

1. serum potassium level of 4
2. hemoglobin of 13
3. serum cholesterol of 180
4. white blood count of 14,000 mm^3

4-23

You are teaching a parent about fever management for a child who has chicken pox. Which of the following treatment modalities is contraindicated?

1. offering plenty of liquids
2. administering aspirin for fever management
3. dressing the child in lightweight clothing
4. teaching the correct technique for using a thermometer

4-24

Who of the following is most likely to experience hepatitis E?

1. an intravenous drug user
2. an immigrant newly arrived from a developing country
3. a toddler in a day-care facility
4. a client receiving hemodialysis

4-25

A client with cancer of the lung is receiving the colony-stimulating factor Filgrastim and is complaining of bone pain. What should you administer to relieve the pain?

1. aspirin 10 gr po
2. acetaminophen 650 mg po
3. meperidine hydrochloride 50 mg intramuscularly
4. morphine sulfate 30 mg po

4-26

A 22-year-old client has Hodgkin's lymphoma. As a consequence of chemotherapy and radiation therapy, the client is immunocompromised. The nurse's aide reported the client's temperature as 100.3°F. The appropriate nursing action is to:

1. retake the temperature after 2 hours.
2. do nothing; a fever is expected in this condition.
3. give the client aspirin 10 gr.
4. notify the physician and prepare to take cultures.

4-27

A 5-year-old with acute lymphocytic leukemia is to be discharged from the hospital in a state of remission. The nurse will reinforce which of the following understandings about the role of the child's parents?

1. Make few demands on the child and try to make the child as happy as possible since the condition is terminal.
2. Guide the child through encouragement and setting limits so that the child may develop full potential.
3. It is not necessary to control the child's behavior since the child's condition will impose limitations.
4. It will be necessary to develop a carefully planned schedule for the child so that energy can be conserved.

4 - 2 8

A client has a laceration approximately 2 inches long and 1 inch deep that has been sustained for approximately 2 hours. You will irrigate the wound with a minimum of:

1. 200 ml of solution.
2. 150 ml of solution.
3. 100 ml of solution.
4. 250 ml of solution.

4 - 2 9

A 4-month-old infant is brought to the clinic for a well-child checkup. Assuming that immunizations are being given as recommended and were begun at 2 months of age, what immunizations should be given at this time?

1. measles, mumps, and rubella vaccine
2. Haemophilus influenzae type B vaccine
3. pneumonia vaccine
4. hepatitis B vaccine

4 - 3 0

A 20-year-old college student is seen in the student health clinic because of fatigue, weight loss, and a low-grade fever. Physical examination reveals slight enlargement of the cervical lymph nodes. Which of the following questions pertaining to the client's fever should the nurse ask initially?

1. "When did you first notice your temperature was elevated?"
2. "Has your temperature been over 102°F?"
3. "Have you recently been exposed to anyone who has an infection?"
4. "Have you had a sore throat?"

4 - 3 1

Your client's enzyme-linked immuno-absorbent assay test was positive. What does this mean?

1. The client is immune to the acquired immunodeficiency syndrome.
2. The client will develop acquired immunodeficiency syndrome in the near future.
3. Antibodies to the human immunodeficiency virus are present in the client's blood.
4. There are no antibodies to the human immunodeficiency virus in the client's blood.

4 - 3 2

A child has acute lymphocytic leukemia. The nurse is planning a room assignment. Which of the following would be the best choice?

1. a private room
2. a room with another child with leukemia
3. a four-bed room with children his age
4. a bed in intensive care

4 - 3 3

Which evidence supports a nursing diagnosis of "high risk for infection related to immuno-deficiency?"

1. decreased leukocyte count
2. decreased serum globulin level
3. increased serum hemoglobin level
4. increased number of T-helper cells

4 - 3 4

A client with acquired immunodeficiency syndrome is receiving the antiviral agent zidovudine. What laboratory studies need to be monitored in the client receiving this medication?

1. serum glutamic-pyruvic transaminase
2. blood urea nitrogen
3. erythrocyte sedimentation rate
4. red blood cell count

4 - 3 5

A client newly diagnosed with hepatitis A should be informed that:

1. this form of hepatitis typically develops into a chronic carrier state.
2. persons who have had hepatitis A have an increased risk for developing liver cancer.
3. hepatitis A is spread only via contaminated serum.
4. the oral-fecal route is the most common cause of the spread of hepatitis A.

4 - 3 6

Your client is at risk for Rh incompatibility. Which client data would support a nursing diagnosis of injury, fetal potential for, related to blood transfusion, for a client at risk for Rh incompatibility?

1. a positive indirect Coombs test
2. a negative direct Coombs test
3. an Rh-positive mother and an Rh-negative father
4. Rhogam given at 28 weeks' gestation

4 - 3 7

The nurse receives a phone call from a mother of 4 children who completed their primary tetanus immunizations 2 years ago. The nurse would need to advise the mother to have a booster dose of tetanus toxoid for which one of her children?

1. the child who sustained scratches on bare legs while climbing on a backyard fence
2. the child who is hospitalized and having emergency treatment for a perforated appendix
3. the child who is having dental treatment for an abscessed impacted molar
4. the child who walked barefoot in the woods and sustained an injury by stepping on a nail

4 - 3 8

The nurse should recognize which of the following factors in a client's history as most likely to be related to hepatitis A?

1. recently recovered from an upper respiratory infection
2. was bitten by an insect
3. had contact with a person who was jaundiced
4. ate home-canned foods

4 - 3 9

A client presents signs and symptoms of malaise, low-grade fever, and fatigue after being exposed to chicken pox 2 weeks earlier. What stage of illness is the client experiencing?

1. incubation
2. prodromal
3. illness
4. convalescence

4 - 4 0

Infection with the human immunodeficiency virus progresses to acquired immuno-deficiency syndrome more quickly in infants. This process is due to:

1. the human immunodeficiency virus attacking the organs of the infant.
2. the infant's immune system being over-taken by the mother's human immuno-deficiency virus antibodies.
3. the human immunodeficiency virus attacking the infant's immune system, which has not formed antibodies.
4. the human immunodeficiency virus attacking the infant's organs during their various stages of development.

4 - 4 1

A client with acquired immunodeficiency syndrome has developed Kaposi's sarcoma. The physician has prescribed interferon Alfa 2b, 30 million units 3 times a week. The following is a teaching plan related to self-administration of interferon. Which of the following information is incorrect and should not be included in the teaching plan?

1. The client can substitute a less expensive generic interferon in place of the one prescribed.
2. Most clients tend to experience flulike symptoms that should diminish with con-tinued therapy.
3. The drug should be administered at bed-time to minimize daytime drowsiness.
4. The client should avoid contact with per-sons with viral illness and those who have recently taken vaccines.

4 - 4 2

Which diagnoses would be given the highest priority for a child with varicella?

1. potential sleep pattern disturbance related to pruritus
2. potential nutritional alteration: less than body requirements related to oral lesions
3. potential for infection related to bacterial invasion of skin lesions
4. impaired social interaction related to isolation during the contagious period

4 - 4 3

To determine if the immune system is functioning adequately, your assessment would reveal:

1. a positive Homans' sign.
2. the absence of fasciculations.
3. a positive Babinski reflex.
4. a positive reaction to skin testing.

4 - 4 4

The nurse is planning care for a client convalescing from the hepatitis A virus. The nurse will expect the client to have the most difficulty:

1. relieving pain.
2. regulating bowel elimination.
3. maintaining a sense of well-being.
4. preventing respiratory complications.

4 - 4 5

You have never had chicken pox and learn that you have been exposed to a client with herpes zoster. Within 96 hours, you should receive:

1. the immune globulin.
2. the varicella-zoster immune globulin.
3. a full course of antibiotic therapy.
4. a Tzanck test to determine herpes.

4 - 4 6

Which of the following should be completed before beginning an anti-infective?

1. Allergies should be identified and the culture specimens collected.
2. The culture report should be on the chart and allergies identified.
3. A history should be taken and the offending organism identified.
4. Allergy tests, a history, and a physical should be completed.

4-47

A 15-year-old client is admitted to the hospital with sickle-cell anemia. The client states, "My knees are killing me. I guess that's why I can't walk to the bathroom and back to bed without getting short of breath." An appropriate nursing response would be to:

1. agree with the client and assist the client back to bed.
2. explain in understandable terms how sickle-cell anemia can affect mobility.
3. administer an analgesic so that the client will be able to walk back to the bed without getting short of breath.
4. explain that the white blood count is high and the client should be careful walking back and forth to the bathroom.

4-48

A client has been given an antibiotic. Which assessment finding indicates this medication has been effective?

1. passage of a formed stool
2. voiding 500 cc over 2 hours
3. a statement that pain is relieved
4. temperature decreasing to 98.6°F

4-49

The physician has requested peak and trough levels in association with tobramycin therapy. The nurse will know that peak and trough levels are used to:

1. determine efficacy of the drug.
2. determine if the client is allergic to the drug.
3. establish and maintain therapeutic serum levels without excessive toxicity.
4. determine the correct therapeutic loading of the initial dose.

4-50

What changes in laboratory studies are seen as the disease process of human immuno-deficiency virus progresses?

1. platelet count increases
2. T-4 lymphocyte count decreases
3. T-8 lymphocyte count decreases
4. erythrocyte sedimentation rate decreases

4 - 5 1

A 7-year-old is diagnosed with typhoid fever. The nurse will:

1. wear gloves due to the infectious materials.
2. wear a mask because the client may have a cough.
3. place the client on strict isolation because the client may have a cough.
4. place the client on contact isolation because of wound infection.

4 - 5 2

The nurse will recognize the first sign of testicular cancer as:

1. the ability to transilluminate the testicle using a penlight.
2. urinary frequency and urgency.
3. lumbar pain.
4. painless enlargement of the testicle.

4 - 5 3

The most common pathogen found in the bladder and upper urinary tract is:

1. *Escherichia coli* (E. coli).
2. *Streptococcus pyogenes* (group A).
3. *Staphylococcus aureus*.
4. *Salmonella*.

4 - 5 4

Which of the following populations would be most likely to test positive for hepatitis D?

1. children who attend an overcrowded day-care facility
2. health-care workers who have received hepatitis C vaccine
3. persons who are diagnosed with hepatitis B
4. anyone in the population

4 - 5 5

A client diagnosed with hepatitis B should be informed that:

1. hepatitis B is spread only via the oral-fecal route.
2. hepatitis B vaccine may be administered only after a person reaches 18 years of age.
3. there is no hepatitis B immune globulin.
4. standard precautions are indicated for all contacts.

4 - 5 6

The nurse provides a client with information about the most common side effects of mechlorethamine hydrochloride and measures that can be used to counteract these side effects. Which of the following measures, if incorporated in the client's nursing-care plan, would diminish the most common side effects of this medication?

1. encouraging high fluid intake
2. providing a diet high in fiber
3. obtaining a prescription for niacin
4. administering a pretreatment antiemetic

4 - 5 7

A client with a history of skin cancer will be advised to use:

1. benzyl benzoate lotion.
2. undecylenic acid powder.
3. desonide ointment.
4. para-aminobenzoic acid lotions.

4 - 5 8

A client with acquired immunodeficiency syndrome has been hospitalized. During your initial assessment of the client, you observe cheesy-looking white patches in the client's mouth. When the patches are rubbed, erythema and bleeding occur. You suspect:

1. herpes simplex.
2. candidiasis.
3. leukoplakia.
4. Kaposi's sarcoma.

4 - 5 9

An appropriate nursing intervention for a client with tetanus is to:

1. decrease environmental stimulation.
2. suction by the nasopharyngeal route.
3. gently massage the large joints.
4. frequently assess the level of consciousness.

4 - 6 0

Your client has experienced a bone marrow biopsy and is complaining of tenderness. You would:

1. administer the prescribed analgesic.
2. notify the physician of the client's complaint.
3. tell the client this is a normal reaction to the biopsy.
4. apply direct pressure to the tender area.

Practice Test 4

Answers, Explanations, and Rationales

4 - 1

④ **The nurse will place sterile towels soaked in sterile saline over the eviscerated wound. An evisceration is the protrusion of visceral organs through a wound opening. The condition is a medical emergency that requires surgical repair. If the organs protrude through the wound, the blood supply to the tissues is compromised. When evisceration occurs, the nurse places sterile towels soaked in sterile saline over the extruding tissues to reduce the possibility of bacterial invasion and drying.**

1. The physician should be notified, but only after the sterile towels soaked in sterile saline have been placed over the wound.

2. Placing an unsterile dry dressing over an evisceration will expose the wound to infection and dry out the wound.

3. Surgery is required and ointment would have to be removed. Also, Betadine should not be placed on the organs because it is an irritant.

Nursing Process: Implementing
Client Need: Safe, Effective Care Environment

4 - 2

③ **A child who has an illness should not receive immunizations. The child's health is already compromised, and immunizations may compromise it further.**

1. A child who has been exposed to an infectious disease but has no symptoms of illness could be immunized.

2. Children who are presently receiving antimicrobial (anti-infective) therapy may receive immunizations.

4. The fact that a child had a moderate local reaction to a previous vaccine injection does not mean that the child is not a candidate for other vaccinations.

Nursing Process: Evaluating
Client Need: Health Promotion and Maintenance

4 - 3

① **Anorexia is the most common early symptom of hepatitis A. Chills, nausea, vomiting, dyspepsia, and tenderness of the liver are other early manifestations of Type A hepatitis. Type A hepatitis is usually spread by the fecal-oral route as a result of poor hygiene or a breakdown in sanitary conditions. Enteric precautions are recommended.**

2, 3, and 4. Abdominal distention, ecchymosis (blue-black hemorrhagic areas of the skin), and shortness of breath are symptoms of advanced liver disease.

Nursing Process: Assessing
Client Need: Physiological Integrity

4 - 4

① The nurse will inform clients receiving chemotherapy that alopecia (hair loss) is temporary and that hair growth will occur soon after chemotherapy is discontinued.

2. Even though alopecia (hair loss) is transient, it is a very traumatic experience for many clients and would be considered more than a minor side effect of chemotherapy.

3. Alopecia (hair loss) cannot be minimized by adjusting the dosage of the causative medication.

4. Alopecia (hair loss) is not permanent. However, the client should be taught that when hair growth returns, the hair could be a different color and texture.

Nursing Process: Implementing

Client Need: Physiological Integrity

4 - 5

③ The nurse will teach the parents that their baby's jaundice is caused by excessive destruction of the red blood cells (RBCs). Hemolytic disease of the newborn (HDN, erythroblastosis fetalis) results from excessive destruction of fetal red blood cells by maternal antibodies. The end product of red blood cell destruction is excessive bilirubin (hyperbilirubinemia), which the infant's immature liver is unable to metabolize. The result is jaundice.

1. Polycythemia (an abnormal, excessive number of red blood cells) is not associated with HDN.

2. Melanin (the pigment that gives skin and hair its color) is not associated with HDN.

4. An infant who has HDN will have hyperbilirubinemia, not hypobilirubinemia.

Nursing Process: Implementing

Client Need: Physiological Integrity

4 - 6

② The nurse's teaching plan for the client should include the need to increase fluid intake. Hemorrhagic cystitis is a common side effect of cyclophosphamide that may be diminished by increasing fluid intake (approximately 3 liters per day).

1 and 3. None of the prescribed medications require a cardiology workup or cause photosensitivity.

4. Nausea will cause clients to have an aversion to foods they like and defeats the goal of good nutrition.

Nursing Process: Planning

Client Need: Physiological Integrity

4 - 7

③ **The nurse will recognize constipation as a common side effect of morphine. Other common side effects of opiates include sedation, nausea, vomiting, and decreased respiratory rate.**

1. Effective pain relief would require minimal rescue doses of medication.
2. Frequent rescue doses indicate underdosage or undertreatment, not a side effect of morphine.
4. The client's pulse rate would increase, not decrease, to compensate for lack of oxygen.

Nursing Process: Evaluating
Client Need: Physiological Integrity

4 - 8

② **The nurse will anticipate separation from family, especially the mother, as the most traumatic event for a hospitalized toddler.**

1, 3, and 4. Inhibition from running about freely; placement in an unfamiliar environment; and disruption of routines and rituals will all require adjustment by the toddler, but are not considered traumatic.

Nursing Process: Analyzing
Client Need: Psychosocial Integrity

4 - 9

③ **The administration of packed red blood cells will be anticipated. Anemia exists when there is a reduction of red blood cells, a decrease in hemoglobin, and a drop in the volume of packed red blood cells. Therapy is aimed at replacing the red blood cells that carry oxygen to the body.**

1. 6.8 gm/dL is not a normal hemoglobin count. The normal hemoglobin count for the female adult is 12 to 16 gm/100 ml. The normal hemoglobin count for the adult male is 14 to 18 gm/100 ml.

2 and 4. The hemoglobin would not be affected by intravenous albumin or normal saline.

Nursing Process: Planning
Client Need: Health Promotion and Maintenance

4-10

③ **The nursing-care plan will include protecting the client from injury. A client with thrombocytopenia (abnormal decrease in the number of blood platelets) should be protected from injury because of the low platelet count. Should the client sustain an injury, abnormal bleeding would occur due to an impaired clotting mechanism.**

1. The immediate concern is to prevent injury and the potential for bleeding. Placing the client in a 45-degree position may facilitate breathing, but positioning is not the major concern.

2. There is no indication that the client should limit fluids.

4. Exercising the client's lower extremities is contraindicated. Nothing should be done that would facilitate bleeding. Soft toothbrushes and electric razors should be used and the client should avoid aspirin.

Nursing Process: Planning
Client Need: Health Promotion and Maintenance

4-11

② **Clients who are experiencing hemarthrosis (bleeding into the cavity of a joint) should have the affected joint immobilized. Immobilization of a joint in a position of slight flexion will prevent bleeding from further trauma.**

1. Passive exercise should not begin until the active phase of the disease has passed.

3. Wrapping the joint in an elastic bandage to apply pressure would not prevent bleeding but may be done to assist in immobilization of the joint.

4. A tourniquet would not prevent bleeding in this case but may cause additional trauma due to restriction of the blood supply.

Nursing Process: Planning
Client Need: Safe, Effective Care Environment

4-12

① **Xerostomia is dryness of the mouth due to an alteration in normal secretions. It is a side effect of some chemotherapies and can be very distressing to clients. It places the client at an increase for infections of the oral cavity.**

2. Alopecia refers to hair loss.

3. Xanthoma is a type of skin lesion.

4. Anemia is a blood disorder whose hallmark is low or abnormal hemoglobin levels.

Nursing Process: Implementing
Client Need: Physiological Integrity

4 - 1 3

④ **The nurse is not likely to observe signs of bleeding such as bruising. Bruising is more likely to indicate bleeding tendencies, especially in fleshy areas. Bleeding tendencies are not common in sickle-cell disease.**

1. Paleness is usually present in clients with sickle-cell anemia because of low hemoglobin levels. Palms of hands and soles of feet are good areas to note skin color in persons with dark pigmentation.

2. Growth retardation of both height and weight is commonly found in children with sickle-cell disease.

3. Increased heart rates help compensate for low hemoglobin levels. Cyanosis is usually not present because most, if not all, hemoglobin in arterial circulation is adequately oxygenated.

Nursing Process: Assessing

Client Need: Physiological Integrity

4 - 1 4

④ **Prior to administering blood, the nurse will verify the prescription and labels carefully with another nurse. Administering incompatible blood by mistake can be a fatal error, causing hemolytic reaction and shock. The companion check system radically reduces the risk of such an error.**

1. Blood transfusions typically last from 1 to 2 hours. If the blood has been refrigerated, it should be given within 30 minutes of the time it was removed from the refrigerator.

2. Antibiotics are not routinely given prior to blood transfusions.

3. Dextrose may hemolyze the blood. Blood can only be administered with normal saline (physiological saline).

Nursing Process: Implementing

Client Need: Health Promotion and Maintenance

4 - 1 5

② **The nurse should teach the parents of a child with rubella not to allow friends or relatives who are pregnant to visit for at least 5 days after the rubella rash disappears. If a pregnant woman is not immune and contracts rubella in her first trimester, the fetus can develop birth defects such as cataracts, heart murmurs, and deafness.**

1. Trying to prevent the child from playing with brothers and sisters until the child no longer has a rash is unrealistic.

3 and 4. The contagious period for rubella is 7 days before the appearance of the rash and 5 days after the appearance of the rash. Therefore, siblings are already exposed.

Nursing Process: Implementing

Client Need: Safe, Effective Care Environment

4 - 1 6

④ **The nurse will advise the client to avoid crowded public situations. Clients with a white blood cell count (WBC) of <2000/cm³ are at an increased risk for contracting infection because their immune systems are compromised. Clients with a low WBC should also be advised to practice frequent handwashing, as should all persons with whom they have contact.**

1. This client is not contagious. The client is at an increased risk for contracting an infection.

2. It is inappropriate to make judgments regarding a client's desire for celebrations. It is therapeutic to maintain a sense of normality during times of change and crisis for clients.

3. There is no indication that this client should avoid carbohydrates. Many clients who are in the midst of chemotherapy suffer from nutritional deficits and efforts should be made to encourage them to enjoy their meals.

Nursing Process: Implementing
Client Need: Health Promotion and Maintenance

4 - 1 7

① **Oral polio vaccine (OPV) is generally considered unsafe to give to an infant whose caregiver may be immunosuppressed because the virus in the oral vaccine is shed in the stool and the caregiver may be exposed to the virus.**

2, 3, and 4. There are no specific contraindications for the intramuscular immunizations for hepatitis B, diphtheria, tetanus, pertussis, or Haemophilus influenzae type B.

Nursing Process: Analyzing
Client Need: Safe, Effective Care Environment

4 - 1 8

② **The nurse should include measures that prevent bleeding and bruising. Platelets help the blood to clot. Clients with low platelet counts, or those less than 150 cells x 109/L, are at risk for spontaneous hemorrhage. Nursing care must be scrupulous in preventing any bruising or bleeding.**

1. A low platelet count is not associated with profound muscle pain.

3 and 4. Both parenteral medication and vigorous range-of-motion exercises should be avoided because of the increased risk for bruising or bleeding.

Nursing Process: Planning
Client Need: Health Promotion and Maintenance

4-19

① The nurse will teach the child's parents that the Haemophilus influenzae type B (HiB) vaccine is given to protect a child from serious infections such as epiglottitis, bacterial pneumonia, bacterial meningitis, and sepsis.

2 and 3. The HiB vaccine does not prevent hepatitis B or human immunodeficiency virus (HIV).

4. HiB is not associated with the virus that causes influenza.

Nursing Process: Implementing
Client Need: Safe, Effective Care Environment

4-20

④ Clients with acute hepatitis B should be advised to avoid contact sports. Hepatitis is a viral infection in the liver that causes the liver to become friable and enlarged. Sudden jarring motions or potential for blows to the abdomen should be avoided in persons experiencing such an infection.

1. An increase in carbohydrates is accepted therapy for persons experiencing viral hepatitis.

2. Clients may sleep in any position of comfort during an illness with hepatitis B.

3. Antihistamines in moderation are appropriate for the pruritus that may occur with the jaundice.

Nursing Process: Implementing
Client Need: Health Promotion and Maintenance

4-21

③ Clients with autoimmune chronic hepatitis will have elevated liver function tests. Autoimmune chronic hepatitis is characterized by chronic inflammation of the liver that is not caused by viruses or toxin ingestion. As implied by the name, it is thought to be autoimmune in its etiology. Liver function tests are typically markedly elevated, as in all the hepatitis variations. Serum bilirubin levels are usually elevated, too. There are also specific titers for some of the antibodies associated with this disorder.

1. Autoimmune chronic hepatitis is not associated with hepatitis B. Unless the two disorders occurred coincidentally, there would be no concurrent elevation of hepatitis B surface antigen in the presence of autoimmune chronic hepatitis.

2 and 4. Liver function and bilirubin levels all tend to be elevated in clients with autoimmune chronic hepatitis.

Nursing Process: Evaluating
Client Need: Physiological Integrity

4-22

④ **A white blood count (WBC) of 14,000 mm³ indicates an infectious process. A normal white blood cell count (WBC) is 4000 to 10,000 mm³.**

1. A normal potassium level is 3.5 to 5.5. Potassium levels are not associated with infection.

2. A normal hemoglobin level is 14 to 18 for men and 12 to 16 for women. Hemoglobin levels are not associated with infection.

3. Cholesterol levels should be less than 200. Therefore, a cholesterol of 180 is within normal limits. Cholesterol levels are not associated with infection.

Nursing Process: Evaluating

Client Need: Physiological Integrity

4-23

② **Aspirin should not be given to children with a viral illness such as chicken pox due to the association between the use of aspirin and Reye syndrome.**

1. Adequate hydration is essential in fever management. Otherwise, a client can easily become dehydrated.

3. Dressing the child in lightweight clothing and exposing the skin to air is an effective means of fever reduction after an antipyretic is administered.

4. Proper temperature assessment is vital when initiating therapeutic interventions.

Nursing Process: Implementing

Client Need: Health Promotion and Maintenance

4-24

② **An immigrant newly arrived from a developing country is most likely to experience hepatitis E. Hepatitis E is virtually unknown in North America. It is one of the viral liver infections spread via the fecal-oral route and is typically found only in developing countries. Hepatitis E should be considered as a possible cause of illness in those persons who have recently traveled to a developing country.**

1. An intravenous drug user is more likely to contract hepatitis B, C, and perhaps D.

3. A toddler in a day-care facility is more likely to contract hepatitis A.

4. Clients receiving hemodialysis are more likely to contract hepatitis B, C, and perhaps D.

Nursing Process: Analyzing

Client Need: Health Promotion and Maintenance

4 - 2 5

② The nurse will administer acetaminophen (Tylenol) 650 mg po. The most common side effect of neupogen (Filgrastim) is bone pain. The pain is readily relieved by nonnarcotic analgesics such as acetaminophen (Tylenol).

1. Clients with bone marrow suppression should avoid aspirin to prevent potential bleeding.

3. Meperidine hydrochloride (Demerol) is an opioid analgesic. However, it is not necessary to administer an opioid when the pain can be relieved by acetaminophen (Tylenol). Also, it is better to give the medication po to prevent bleeding.

4. Morphine sulfate (Astramorph) is an opioid analgesic. However, it is not necessary to administer an opioid when the pain can be relieved by acetaminophen (Tylenol).

Nursing Process: Implementing

Client Need: Physiological Integrity

4 - 2 6

④ The appropriate nursing action is to notify the physician and prepare to take cultures.

1. A client with a body temperature of 100.3°F should be monitored more frequently than every 2 hours. Also, there is no reason to think that the temperature will subside with the passing of time unless treatment is begun.

2. A body temperature of 100.3°F is not normal. It may be expected since the client's immune system is compromised; however, treatment should be begun to prevent further compromise of the client's health.

3. Giving aspirin is contraindicated because immunosuppression lowers the platelet count and aspirin would increase the risk of gastrointestinal bleeding. Acetaminophen (Tylenol) is the drug of choice. Aspirin would only mask the symptoms. Since the client's immune system is compromised, there is a need to identify the causative organism.

Nursing Process: Implementing

Client Need: Physiological Integrity

4 - 2 7

② The nurse will support the parents as they guide, set limits, and encourage their child.

1. A child with acute lymphocytic leukemia has a greater than 90% chance of achieving an initial remission and approximately one-third may be cured if treated for 30 months.

3. The child is in remission and will need discipline from parents. During remission, the child will not be limited by the condition.

4. During remission, the child will not need a carefully planned schedule that focuses on conservation of energy.

Nursing Process: Implementing

Client Need: Psychosocial Integrity

4-28

④ The nurse will irrigate the wound with a minimum of 250 ml of solution. Generally, wounds are irrigated with 50 ml of solution per 1 inch of the depth and length for each hour.

1, 2, and 3. These amounts of solution are not enough.

Nursing Process: Implementing
Client Need: Health Promotion and Maintenance

4-29

② The infant should receive the Haemophilus influenzae B vaccine at this time. The Haemophilus influenzae B (HiB) vaccine is available for the general public against the Haemophilus influenzae bacteria. There are several formulations of the HiB vaccine. The Pedvax HiB is administered at 2 and 4 months with a booster at 12 months. The HiB-Titer or HbOC is given at 2, 4, and 6 months of age with a booster at 15 months.

1. Measles, mumps, and rubella vaccine (MMR) is given at 15 months and once during childhood.

3. The vaccine against streptococcus pneumonia is recommended for children of 2 years and older who have sickle-cell disease, human immunodeficiency virus, nephrotic syndrome, or Hodgkin's disease.

4. The hepatitis B vaccine is administered within 12 hours of birth, with second and third doses at 1 and 6 months.

Nursing Process: Implementing
Client Need: Health Promotion and Maintenance

4-30

① The nurse should determine when the client first noticed an elevation in temperature. In an attempt to clarify the etiology of the fever, determining when the fever first occurred would be the most appropriate initial question.

2. The elevation of the fever is not as important in determing the etiology of the fever as knowing when the fever was first noted.

3. Infection is only one cause for a fever. Knowing when the fever first occurred would be the best initial question. Also, a question about exposure to infection does not directly relate to fever.

4. A sore throat may or may not be directly related to the fever experienced by the client.

Nursing Process: Assessing
Client Need: Physiological Integrity

4 - 3 1

③ The enzyme-linked immunoabsorbent assay (ELISA) test determines the presence of antibodies directed specifically against the human immunodeficiency virus. The ELISA test does not establish a diagnosis of acquired immunodeficiency syndrome, but does indicate that an individual has been exposed to or infected with the human immunodeficiency virus.

1. There is no known immunity to the human immunodeficiency virus (HIV) that causes acquired immunodeficiency syndrome (AIDS).

2. Determining that a client is infected with or has been exposed to the human immunodeficiency virus should not be interpreted to mean that the client will develop acquired immunodeficiency syndrome (AIDS) in the near future.

4. Having a positive enzyme-linked immunoabsorbent assay (ELISA) test confirms the presence of the antibody associated with the human immunodeficiency virus (HIV).

Nursing Process: Analyzing
Client Need: Physiological Integrity

4 - 3 2

① In planning a room assignment for a child with acute lymphocytic leukemia, the nurse's best choice would be a private room.

2 and 3. Neutropenia (an abnormally small number of neutrophils) predisposes clients with acute lymphocytic leukemia to infection; therefore, placing them in a room with other sick children could be potentially life threatening.

4. Unless the child is critically ill, the intensive care unit would be inappropriate. Until the degree of involvement is determined, a private room is the safest.

Nursing Process: Planning
Client Need: Safe, Effective Care Environment

4 - 3 3

① The data that supports a nursing diagnosis of "high risk for infection related to immunodeficiency" is a decreased leukocyte count.

2, 3, and 4. Clients with immunodeficiency will have an increased serum globulin level, a decreased serum hemoglobin level, and a decreased number of T-helper cells.

Nursing Process: Analyzing
Client Need: Physiological Integrity

4 - 3 4

④ **Persons experiencing acquired immunodeficiency syndrome (AIDS) who receive zidovudine (AZT) should have their red blood count monitored. AZT can be very toxic to bone marrow, producing dose-limiting anemia and neutropenia.**

1. Serum glutamic-pyruvic transaminase (SGPT) tests would be appropriate in diagnosing liver disease and the presence of myocardial infarction.

2. The test for blood urea and nitrogen (BUN) gives an indication of glomerular function and the production and excretion of urea.

3. The erythrocyte sedimentation rate (ESR) test provides information about the inflammatory process in conditions such as rheumatic fever and rheumatic arthritis.

Nursing Process: Evaluating

Client Need: Health Promotion and Maintenance

4 - 3 5

④ **A client newly diagnosed with hepatitis A should be informed that the hepatitis A virus is spread via the oral-fecal route and parenterally. It is found in food and water. Hepatitis A is a viral infection of the liver most commonly found in crowded areas and where food is handled, such as restaurants, schools, day-care centers, and homeless shelters.**

1. Hepatitis A is not associated with a chronic carrier state.

2. Hepatitis A is not associated with an increased risk for developing liver cancer.

3. Hepatitis A may be spread via contaminated serum, but is more commonly spread via the oral-fecal route.

Nursing Process: Implementing

Client Need: Health Promotion and Maintenance

4 - 3 6

① **A positive indirect Coombs test would support a nursing diagnosis of injury, fetal potential for, related to blood transfusion, for a client at risk for Rh incompatibility. A positive Coombs test indicates fetal antigens on maternal cells.**

2. A negative direct Coombs test indicates absence of maternal antibodies on fetal cells.

3. Rh-negative incompatibility requires an Rh-negative mother who is carrying an Rh-positive fetus.

4. Rhogam given at 28 weeks' gestation will not cause injury.

Nursing Process: Assessing

Client Need: Health Promotion and Maintenance

4 - 3 7

④ **The nurse would advise the mother to have a booster dose of tetanus toxoid for the child who stepped on a nail when walking barefoot in the woods. Even though all the children's immunizations are up-to-date, the child who walked barefoot in the woods and sustained an injury by stepping on a nail would have a need for a booster dose of tetanus toxoid. This child sustained an injury in an environment (dirt) where the causative organism (*Clostridium tetani*) is found. *Clostridium tetani* is able to grow in an anaerobic state at the site of the wound.**

1. Sustaining scratches on the legs when climbing a backyard fence is unlikely to expose a child to the *Clostridium tetani* organism.

2. A perforated appendix would not expose a child to the *Clostridium tetani* organism.

3. Dental treatments would not expose a child to the *Clostridium tetani* organism.

Nursing Process: Analyzing
Client Need: Health Promotion and Maintenance

4 - 3 8

③ **The nurse will associate contact with a jaundiced person as a likely factor in acquiring hepatitis A. The hepatitis A virus (HAV) may appear sporadically and can occur from close contact with infected persons. The disease is usually spread by the fecal-oral route. It is often associated with overcrowding, poor hygiene, or breakdown of normal sanitary conditions and may occur in small or large epidemics.**

1. Recent recovery from an upper respiratory infection is not associated with hepatitis A. Hepatitis A is usually spread from person to person via the fecal-oral route and from consuming water contaminated with the hepatitis A virus (HAV).

2. Hepatitis A is not spread via the bite of insects.

4. Consuming home-canned foods would not expose a person to hepatitis A. However, improperly processed foods would expose people to *Clostridium botulinum*.

Nursing Process: Analyzing
Client Need: Physiological Integrity

4 - 3 9

② **A client who has been exposed to chicken pox and has a low-grade fever and fatigue is experiencing the prodromal state of that condition. The prodromal stage is the interval from onset of nonspecific signs and symptoms to the more specific symptoms associated with a condition.**

1. The incubation period is the period of time between exposure to an infection and the appearance of the first symptom of the condition.

3. An illness is the experience of the specific symptoms of a condition such as those associated with tuberculosis, measles, or hepatitis.

4. Convalescence is a period following an illness or an injury during which a client recovers.

Nursing Process: Assessing
Client Need: Physiological Integrity

4 - 4 0

③ **The human immunodeficiency virus (HIV)progresses to acquired immunodeficiency syndrome (AIDS) more quickly in infants because the infant's immune system has not formed antibodies. Within a short period of time (as early as 2 months), the infant develops symptoms of acquired immunodeficiency syndrome (AIDS).**

1. The HIV virus doesn't attack the organs of the infant.

2. The infant's immune system does not receive the mother's HIV antibodies.

4. The HIV virus that causes AIDS does not attack the infant's organs during their various stages of development.

Nursing Process: Evaluating
Client Need: Physiological Integrity

4 - 4 1

① **The care plan should not include the recommendation that the client substitute a less expensive generic interferon. Different brands of interferon (Intron-A) cannot be interchanged due to equivalency and dosage difference.**

2. Clients taking interferon Alfa-2b (Intron-A) will initially experience flulike symptoms. These symptoms usually diminish with continued use.

3. Since interferon Alfa-2b can cause drowsiness, it is helpful to have the client take the medication at bedtime.

4. Since the client's immune system is compromised, it is not recommended that the client be in contact with persons with viral illnesses.

Nursing Process: Planning
Client Need: Health Promotion and Maintenance

4 - 4 2

③ **The diagnosis with the highest priority for a child with varicella (chicken pox) is a potential for infection related to bacterial invasion of skin lesions. Secondary bacterial infections are common complications since children are likely to scratch the lesions.**

1, 2, and 4. Sleep pattern disturbances related to pruritus; nutrition alteration related to oral lesions; and impaired social interaction related to isolation are short-term discomforts and would not be the nursing diagnosis with the highest priority.

Nursing Process: Analyzing
Client Need: Health Promotion and Maintenance

4 - 4 3

④ **The nurse can determine if a client's immune system is functioning properly if the client has a positive reaction to a skin test after exposure to a disease such as tuberculosis. For example, if a client has been exposed to the tubercle bacillus or has an active case of tuberculosis, the client should have a positive reaction to the purified protein derivation (PPD) skin test.**

1. A positive Homans' sign is indicative of phlebitis.

2. Absence of fasciculations does not relate to the immune system. (Fasciculation refers to involuntary contractions or twitching of muscle fibers).

3. A positive Babinski reflex is indicative of an upper motor neuron disorder and is not associated with the proper functioning of the immune system.

Nursing Process: Assessing
Client Need: Physiological Integrity

4 - 4 4

③ **The nurse will expect clients recovering from hepatitis A to have difficulty maintaining a sense of well-being. The recovery is slow and clients may continue to have anorexia, malaise, and irritability. It is important for the nurse to work with these clients and their families during the course of the recovery.**

1. Clients experiencing hepatitis A virus (HAV) may experience vague epigastric distress, nausea, heartburn, and flatulence. During the icteric phase (jaundice), the client may experience tenderness of the liver. However, relieving pain is not expected to be a problem.

2. Bowel elimination is not a concern during the convalescent period.

4. Mild flulike upper respiratory tract infection is seen when symptoms first appear. However, respiratory complications are not a concern during convalescence.

Nursing Process: Implementing
Client Need: Health Promotion and Maintenance

4 - 4 5

② For persons who are susceptible, the varicella-zoster immune globulin should be given within 96 hours of exposure. The infection of herpes zoster is contagious until the crusts have dried and fallen off the skin.

1. Immune globulin is used for prophylaxis of measles, hepatitis A, and for the treatment of hypogammaglobulinemia in immunodeficient clients.

3. Herpes zoster is an acute infectious disease caused by the varicella-zoster virus. Therefore, antibiotics are not effective in treating this condition.

4. A Tzanck test consists of examining tissue from the lower surface of a lesion in a vesicular condition to determine the cell type. The Tzanck smear is not associated with immunity from the varicella-zoster virus.

Nursing Process: Implementing
Client Need: Safe, Effective Care Environment

4 - 4 6

① Before administering anti-infective therapy, a client's allergies should be identified and culture specimens should be collected. It is important to know a client's allergies so that allergic reactions such as anaphylaxis can be avoided. Also, before the anti-infective therapy is begun, culture specimens should be collected.

2. You do not need to wait until the culture report is actually in the client's chart to begin anti-infective therapy.

3. The organism does not need to be identified before an anti-infective therapy can be started. A physical and history can provide enough information to administer anti-infective therapy.

4. Allergy tests are not usually necessary prior to administering anti-infective therapy. A client's history is usually sufficient.

Nursing Process: Planning
Client Need: Safe, Effective Care Environment

4 - 4 7

② **An appropriate nursing response would include in understandable terms how sickle-cell anemia can affect mobility. The client should understand that activity intolerance between oxygen supply and demand is associated with shortness of breath, not the pain the client is experiencing in the knees.**

1. One of the primary responsibilities of a nurse is client education. A client with sickle-cell anemia should be taught that pain is caused by a lack of oxygen to the tissues due to low hemoglobin.

3. An analgesic will not prevent the client from becoming short of breath.

4. An abnormally high white blood cell count does not cause shortness of breath. An abnormally low red blood cell count would cause shortness of breath.

Nursing Process: Implementing
Client Need: Physiological Integrity

4 - 4 8

④ **If the antibiotic is effective against infection, the temperature should return to normal. Antibiotics inhibit the growth or destroy microorganisms. A person's temperature becomes elevated in response to infection.**

1. A laxative or stool softener would facilitate the passage of a formed stool.

2. A diuretic would increase fluid volume by increasing urine output.

3. An analgesic would relieve pain.

Nursing Process: Evaluating
Client Need: Physiological Integrity

4 - 4 9

③ **The nurse will know that establishing a peak and trough level for a medication means to establish and maintain therapeutic serum levels without excessive toxicity.**

1. The efficacy of medications such as the anti-infectant tobramycin (Tobrex) is determined by relief of symptoms. Tobramycin's bactericidal action against susceptible bacteria relieves symptoms of infections including bone infections, central nervous system infections (CNS), respiratory infections, septicemia, and endocarditis.

2. Allergies are not associated with peak and trough levels. Allergies should be determined before medications are administered.

4. The initial loading dose of tobramycin is determined by factors that include client body weight. All doses after the initial loading dose are determined by renal function/blood levels, since tobramycin is nephrotoxic.

Nursing Process: Evaluating
Client Need: Physiological Integrity

4 - 5 0

② **As the effects of the human immunodeficiency virus (HIV) progress, the T-4 lymphocyte count decreases. Other laboratory changes include anemia, increased sedimentation rate, thrombocytopenia, and increased levels of B2 macroglobulin.**

1. Decreases in platelet counts occur after HIV has progressed to the point of attacking the bone marrow. This does not occur in all clients who have HIV.

3. The T-8 lymphocyte count remains unchanged but the ratio of T-4 cells to T-8 cells gradually reverses.

4. The erythrocyte sedimentation rate (ESR) increases as HIV disease progresses.

Nursing Process: Evaluating

Client Need: Health Promotion and Maintenance

4 - 5 1

① **The nurse caring for a client with typhoid fever should wear gloves due to infectious materials. The causative organism for typhoid fever is *Salmonella typhus*. The source of *Salmonella typhus* is contaminated water, food, infected urine, and feces (fecal carrier most common source). The control is through vaccinations, establishment of sanitary conditions, good handwashing, treatment and control of carriers, pasteurized milk and dairy products, and sanitary disposition of human feces.**

2. A mask is not required since typhoid fever is not transmitted via the respiratory tract.

3. Typhoid fever does not require strict or contact isolation.

4. The client is not placed on contact isolation because of wound infection. Clients with typhoid fever require enteric precautions. The nurse should observe standard precautions. Contact isolation is instituted for conditions such as acute respiratory infections, herpes, and wound infections.

Nursing Process: Implementing

Client Need: Safe, Effective Care Environment

4 - 5 2

④ **The nurse will recognize the first signs of testicular cancer as painless enlargement of the testicle. Another early sign includes "heaviness" of the scrotum.**

1. If blood or tissue is present in the testicle, transillumination cannot be accomplished.

2. Urgency and urinary frequency are seen in more advanced stages of testicular cancer.

3. Lumbar pain is a sign seen in more advanced stages of testicular cancer and is usually due to metastasis.

Nursing Process: Assessing

Client Need: Health Promotion and Maintenance

4 - 5 3

① *Escherichia coli (E. coli)* is the most common pathogenic organism found in the bladder and upper urinary tract.

2. *Streptococcus pyogenes* (group A) is found in the nasopharynx (upper respiratory tract), on the skin, hair, and perianal area.

3. *Staphylococcus aureus* is found on the skin, hair, and perianal area along with *Streptococcus pyogenes* (group A).

4. Salmonella is found in the small bowel and colon.

Nursing Process: Analyzing

Client Need: Safe, Effective Care Environment

4 - 5 4

③ **The most likely persons to test positive for hepatitis D are those diagnosed with hepatitis B. Hepatitis D is a viral superinfection that occurs only in the presence of hepatitis B. It is thought to be spread in the same manner as hepatitis B but requires the helper function of hepatitis B for its expression. Only persons with hepatitis B may contract hepatitis D.**

1. Children attending an overcrowded day-care facility are at risk for developing hepatitis A, which is spread via the oral-fecal route and is found in food and water.

2. There is no vaccine for hepatitis C.

4. Hepatitis D can only be found in persons who experience hepatitis B.

Nursing Process: Evaluating

Client Need: Safe, Effective Care Environment

4 - 5 5

④ **A client diagnosed with hepatitis B should be informed that standard precautions are indicated for all contacts. Hepatitis B is spread via body fluids. The antigen (virus) is found in serum, saliva, stool, semen, and urine. All body fluids are to be treated as contaminated and universal or standard precautions must be taken at home.**

1. Hepatitis B is spread via body fluids such as serum, saliva, stool, semen, and urine.

2 and 3. Hepatitis B vaccine may be administered to individuals as young as 24 hours old. There is a hepatitis B immune globulin that should be administered as soon as possible after an exposure to the virus.

Nursing Process: Implementing

Client Need: Safe, Effective Care Environment

4 - 5 6

④ **Administration of a pretreatment antiemetic would diminish the most common side effect of mechlorethamine hydrochloride (Mustargen). Mustargen is an antineoplastic (alkylating agent). One of the most common side effects of Mustargen is nausea and vomiting. Administration of pretreatment antiemetics should be completed 30 minutes before Mustargen is administered. Acute toxic signs include nausea and vomiting lasting 12 to 24 hours.**

1 and 2. A high-fluid and high-fiber diet is not recommended. However, the diet should be adjusted so that it is tolerated by the client. This will help to maintain fluid and electrolyte balance as well as good nutrition.

3. Niacin is a lipid-lowering agent administered to treat clients with pellagra and hyperlipemia.

Nursing Process: Planning

Client Need: Physiological Integrity

4 - 5 7

④ **Clients who have experienced skin cancer are advised to protect their skin from ultraviolet radiation by covering their skin with clothing or using a sunscreen. Para-aminobenzoic acid (PABA) is an ingredient in many products that effectively screens out the harmful ultraviolet effects of the sun.**

1. Benzyl benzoate (Scabanca) lotion is used to treat scabies.

2. Undecylenic acid (Desenex powder) is an antifungal.

3. Desonide (Tridesilon) ointment is a topical corticosteroid that does not have an impact on skin cancer.

Nursing Process: Implementing

Client Need: Health Promotion and Maintenance

4 - 5 8

② **You will suspect candidiasis. Candidiasis (thrush) appears as cheesy white patches that, when rubbed, cause erythema (redness of mucosa) and bleeding. Predisposing factors include immunosuppression.**

1. Herpes simplex appears as a singular vesicle or clustered vesicles that usually occur where the mucous membrane joins the skin. It is an opportunistic viral infection (an infection or disease caused by an organism that does not normally cause disease except under certain circumstances, such as in immunosuppressed clients).

3. Leukoplakia is a disease affecting the mucous membranes of the cheeks, gums, and tongue. It appears as white thick patches that have a tendency to fissure (cleft or furrow). Leukoplakia is associated with use of tobacco and poorly fitted dentures.

4. Kaposi's sarcoma appears first on the oral mucosa as a reddish, purple, or blue malignant lesion. Lesions may be singular or multiple in number. Kaposi's sarcoma is an opportunistic neoplasm affecting clients with acquired immunodeficiency syndrome (AIDS).

Nursing Process: Assessing
Client Need: Physiological Integrity

4 - 5 9

① **An appropriate nursing intervention for a client with tetanus (lockjaw) would be to decrease environmental stimuli. Stimulation of these clients causes severe muscle spasms without loss of consciousness. Although strong sedation and muscle relaxants are usually administered, care should be exercised to avoid unnecessary stimulation.**

2. Suctioning by the nasopharyngeal route would be too stimulating and is not necessary since there are no excess secretions.

3. Gentle massage to the large joints may be too stimulating. The discomfort of tetanus is felt more in the muscles than in the joints.

4. Frequent assessment is not necessary since the level of consciousness (LOC) is not affected by tetanus.

Nursing Process: Implementing
Client Need: Safe, Effective Care Environment

4-60

① **A client experiencing tenderness following a bone marrow biopsy would receive the prescribed analgesic. Tenderness is expected following a bone marrow biopsy. Administering the prescribed analgesics will usually resolve the problem.**

2. If tenderness is accompanied by other signs of infection, it would be appropriate to notify the physician.

3. Because tenderness is a normal expectation, an analgesic is anticipated.

4. Applying direct pressure will probably increase the tenderness and is not recommended.

Nursing Process: Implementing

Client Need: Safe, Effective Care Environment

Practice Test 5

Integumentary Systems and Burns

5 - 1

A child sustains deep partial-thickness burns to the arms and anterior chest. It has been 8 hours since admission. All of the following are assessment findings at this time. Which one of the following should have the highest priority for intervention?

1. urine output decreased
2. increased restlessness and irritability
3. radial pulses are less palpable
4. hoarseness and stridor

5 - 2

A 5-year-old was hospitalized promptly after sustaining third-degree burns on the anterior chest, upper arms, forearms, and hands. Intravenous infusion was begun, an indwelling urethral catheter inserted, and pressure dressings applied to burned areas. While performing a nursing assessment of the client, which of the following would be most indicative of the need to implement nursing measures to counteract the effects of shock?

1. restlessness and bradycardia
2. air hunger and hyperreflexia
3. intense pain and convulsions
4. pale, clammy skin and thirst

5 - 3

A 6-year-old child has sustained third-degree burns. To plan for the need for fluid replacement, the nurse will consider which of the following?

1. The younger the child, the greater the volume of fluid needed in proportion to body weight.
2. The proportion of body weight contributed by water is smaller during early childhood than it is during adulthood.
3. The fluid needs per kilogram of body weight are variable until the kidneys become functionally more mature at adolescence.
4. The total volume of extracellular fluid per kilogram of body weight increases gradually from birth to adolescence and then stabilizes at the adult level.

5 - 4

You are irrigating a draining wound with sterile saline solution. Which of the following would be the most appropriate procedure to follow?

1. Wash hands, don clean gloves, remove soiled dressing, wash hands, prepare sterile field, don sterile gloves.
2. Prepare sterile field, put on sterile gloves, and remove soiled dressing.
3. Pour solution, wash hands, and remove soiled dressing.
4. Remove soiled dressing, flush wound, and wash hands.

5 - 5

An infant has some localized scaling and red areas on the cheeks, neck, and elbows that are diagnosed as atopic dermatitis. Which of the following instructions regarding the infant's care is most important for the nurse to reinforce for the mother?

1. Bathe the infant daily with a mild soap.
2. Keep the infant's nails cut short.
3. Use only short-sleeved clothing for the infant.
4. Have the other children in the family avoid contact with the infant.

5 - 6

A client experiencing acne vulgaris may benefit from a prescription for:

1. amphotericin B cream.
2. butoconazole nitrate cream.
3. ciclopirox olamine cream.
4. benzoyl peroxide cream.

5 - 7

A client involved in an industrial accident that involved exposure to a gasoline fire is complaining of painful burns to the feet, but denies pain in the burned legs. The nurse will:

1. remove the footwear to assess the feet only, leaving the rest of the clothing intact.
2. keep the client fully clothed to avoid chilling.
3. remove all clothing, then cover the client in a clean sheet.
4. remove footwear and immediately cover the client's feet in antibiotic ointment.

5 - 8

A client who has experienced 25% body surface second-degree burns may require analgesia with:

1. acetaminophen.
2. morphine sulfate.
3. ibuprofen.
4. a transcutaneous electrical nerve stimulator unit.

5 - 9

A client who has experienced deep partial-thickness burns to the left forearm will require which of the following interventions?

1. casting of the left arm to immobilize the elbow and wrist joints
2. antifungal cream bid to affected area for 10 days
3. immediate surgical intervention of the left arm to restore the skin's integrity
4. a tetanus prophylaxis injection if the client's last one was 12 years ago

5 - 1 0

A client has experienced extensive burns and is scheduled for daily hydrotherapy. The chief purpose of hydrotherapy is to:

1. prevent infection.
2. restore fluid balance.
3. maintain wound sterility.
4. remove loose tissue and debris.

5 - 1 1

Two weeks after a skin graft, a client is concerned about the possibility of scarring at the donor site. Which of the following responses by the nurse concerning the care of the donor site would be most appropriate?

1. "Clean the area with soap and water every day and leave it alone."
2. "Apply hydrogen peroxide to the area several times a day."
3. "Use an antibacterial soap and keep the area covered."
4. "Keep the area soft with lanolin cream or lotion."

5 - 1 2

You are to administer a tepid sponge bath to a client with an elevated temperature. To achieve the desired outcome of this procedure, which of the following measures should be used?

1. Stroke the client's skin to cause friction.
2. Give fluids to drink.
3. Allow moisture on the skin to evaporate.
4. Lower the temperature of the room.

5 - 1 3

A client has been diagnosed with Hansen's disease. The nurse will recognize the pharmacologic treatment for this condition as:

1. rifampin and dapsone.
2. amphotericin B and nystatin.
3. cicloprirox and haloprogin.
4. miconazole and clotrimazole.

5 - 1 4

Which of the following medications would be appropriate to administer one-half hour prior to the debridement of a full-thickness burn?

1. acetaminophen
2. fluoxetine
3. meperidine
4. captopril

5 - 1 5

Which intravenous fluid and rate would be most appropriate to administer immediately to an adult with a full-thickness burn on 18% of the body?

1. keep the vein open with normal saline
2. lidocaine (20 to 50 mcg/kg per min) infusion up to 200 to 300 mg in 1 hour
3. keep the vein open with dextrose 5% in water
4. lactated Ringer's solution at 250 cc per hour

5 - 16

A client who had abdominal surgery has a wound drain in place. On the evening following surgery, the dressing covering the incision is saturated with a large quantity of blood-tinged drainage. Which of the following interpetations and actions is most accurate?

1. Hemorrhage is occurring and the physician should be notified.
2. Wound dehiscence is imminent and a firm binder should be applied.
3. This drainage is expected and the dressing should be reinforced.
4. The drain is obstructed and it should be irrigated before the dressing is changed.

5 - 17

Your client is extremely edematous. Which of the following nursing interventions is most appropriate?

1. Cough and deep breathe every 2 hours.
2. Massage extremities with lotion every 4 hours.
3. Turn and reposition every 1 to 2 hours.
4. Place lamb's wool the full length of the bed.

5 - 18

A client is admitted to the Emergency Department with partial- and full-thickness burns on the chest, arms, and hands. On arrival at the emergency facility, which of the following will the nurse anticipate as an immediate action?

1. arterial blood gases
2. morphine sulfate to be given intra-muscularly
3. assessment of the client's home environment
4. body weight assessment

5 - 19

A client who has experienced a "sunburn" after 2 hours of unprotected exposure to the summer's sun most likely has:

1. a superficial partial-thickness burn.
2. a deep partial-thickness burn.
3. a full-thickness burn.
4. no real thermal burn. "Sunburn" is merely a lay term.

5-20

A client experienced extensive burns. What is the first consequence of capillary permeability in the surrounding tissues?

1. fluid loss
2. pain
3. edema
4. nausea

5-21

A child was admitted with burns over 30% of the body due to clothes catching fire. It is now 24 hours later. The lowest priority data to collect at this time is:

1. body weight
2. bowel sounds
3. breath sounds
4. vital signs

5-22

According to the "rule of nines," burn victims experiencing burns to their anterior chest and abdomen have an injury that approximates:

1. 8% of their body's surface.
2. 18% of their body's surface.
3. 29% of their body's surface.
4. above 29% of their body's surface.

5-23

Which of the following will you remove in order to reduce sources of heat in a thermally burned client?

1. jewelry
2. dentures
3. makeup
4. hairpieces

5-24

Clients experiencing fungal skin infections should be advised to avoid using:

1. detergents.
2. cornstarch.
3. cotton clothing.
4. topical creams.

5 - 2 5

A client was recently placed on a regimen of prednisone for severe contact dermatitis. Which of the following instructions should be given to the client?

1. "Take a tablet only when the itch gets really bad."
2. "Make sure you drink a big glass of orange juice with each dose."
3. "Save any leftover pills and take them the next time you get poison oak."
4. "Don't stop taking this medicine abruptly; the dosage must be tapered."

5 - 2 6

An adolescent is experiencing severe acne caused by the microorganism *P. acnes*. Which pharmacological agent is administered to treat this condition?

1. Tetracycline
2. Pyrimethamine
3. Miconazole
4. Famciclovir

5 - 2 7

A client has anemia and is experiencing the following integumentary changes: pallor, jaundice, and pruritus. The nurse knows that pruritus occurs as a result of:

1. reduced hemoglobin and decreased blood flow to the skin.
2. increased serum and skin bile salt concentration.
3. increased concentration of serum bilirubin that increases red blood cell hemolysis.
4. low viscosity of blood.

5 - 2 8

Parents of pediatric clients with chicken pox should be advised to avoid administering:

1. calamine lotion over or around lesions.
2. acetaminophen po for pain.
3. diphenhydramine po for itch.
4. diphenhydramine ointment liberally over the entire body.

5-29

Your client received a partial-thickness (first-degree) burn. You know this degree of burn affects the:

1. epidermis.
2. epidermis and dermis.
3. epidermis, dermis, and subcutaneous tissue.
4. skin and nerve endings.

5-30

A 4-year-old is experiencing cellulitis of the right forearm. There is swelling above the wrist and beyond the elbow. You will teach the caregiver how to use:

1. elastic bandages to reduce swelling.
2. elbow restraints for immobilization.
3. warm, moist compresses.
4. range-of-motion exercise to prevent contracture.

5-31

A client with condylomata acuminata has been treating the growths with a self-application of the topical medication podofilox. The client tells the nurse, "I just learned that I am pregnant. Will this interfere with my medication?" The nurse's best response is:

1. "The medication is contraindicated during pregnancy."
2. "It will be necessary to change the route of administration."
3. "There is no reason the medication can't be continued as usual."
4. "Treating the growths now will prevent complications for the baby during delivery."

5-32

You are teaching the parents of a child with impetigo how to treat the child's lesions. Which statement made by the parents indicates a need for further teaching?

1. "We will wash and soak the lesions with warm soapy water 3 times a day."
2. "We will gently remove the crusts after soaking."
3. "We will apply the prescribed topical antibiotic ointment to the affected areas."
4. "We will cover the affected areas with sterile gauze pads."

5 - 3 3

A 7-year-old child has pediculosis capitis. The medication permethrin 1% has been prescribed. The nurse will teach the parents how to administer this topical liquid medication. Which comment by the parents indicates a need for further teaching?

1. "We will apply the medication after our child's hair has been washed with shampoo, rinsed, and towel-dried."
2. "We will apply about 35 ml of the liquid medication to saturate our child's hair and scalp."
3. "We will allow the medication to remain on our child's hair and scalp for 10 minutes before rinsing it off with water."
4. "We will administer a second application of the medication 7 to 10 days after the first application."

5 - 3 4

A client is experiencing vitiligo. This condition is best described as:

1. raised, firm, thickened scabs that form at the site of a wound.
2. ingrown hairs producing papules, pustules, and occasional keloids.
3. unpigmented skin patches.
4. a fungal infection producing yellow- or fawn-colored patches on the skin.

5 - 3 5

A 4-year-old has recently had an autograft following a burn on the anterior chest. Your plan of care is least likely to include:

1. maintaining the client in a supine position.
2. hydrotherapy to stimulate circulation.
3. use of elbow restraints.
4. aspiration of fluid accumulated under the graft.

5 - 3 6

What would you expect your assessment to reveal in a postburn client during the early stages of shock?

1. restlessness
2. marked decrease in blood pressure
3. shallow respirations
4. decrease in urinary output

5-37

A preterm neonate weighing 1,430 grams is under a radiant warmer for phototherapy. The most appropriate nursing diagnosis for this neonate is:

1. skin integrity impaired.
2. gas exchange impaired.
3. fluid volume deficit, potential for.
4. infection, potential for.

5-38

Warm, moist packs have been prescribed qid to treat an ulceration on a client's foot. Aseptic technique will be used to:

1. destroy bacteria on the skin.
2. inhibit the growth of pathogens.
3. prevent the introduction of additional microorganisms.
4. minimize the risk of spreading the infection to others.

5-39

Which of the following is not associated with congenital anomaly?

1. Mongolian spotting over the buttocks
2. short stature, low posterior hairline, webbing of the neck, broad chest, and widely spaced nipples
3. a simian crease across the palms of both hands
4. the top of the pinna falling below an imaginary line from the outer orbit of the eye to the occiput

5-40

A dark-skinned person is experiencing erythema. You will expect the skin to appear:

1. pale.
2. dusky red or violet.
3. black.
4. yellow.

Practice Test 5

Answers, Rationales, and Explanations

5 - 1

④ **Hoarseness and stridor are assessment findings that have the highest priority for intervention at this time. These findings are likely indications of airway edema that is potentially life threatening.**

1, 2, and 3. A decrease in urine output, increased restlessness and irritability, and less palpable radial pulses would not take precedence over potential airway obstruction.

Nursing Process: Analyzing
Client Need: Physiological Integrity

5 - 2

④ **Pale, clammy skin and thirst indicate a need to implement nursing measures to counteract the effects of shock. Burns result in an initial fluid loss due to diuresis and increased capillary permeability.**

1. Initial signs of shock include tachycardia, not bradycardia.

2. Air hunger is associated with a decrease in hemoglobin, not dehydration. Also, the burned client is most likely to experience hyponatremia (sodium depletion), not hypernatremia, which would cause increased muscle tone and deep tendon reflexes.

3. Intense pain and convulsions would be associated with the actual burn, especially painful, deep second-degree burns.

Nursing Process: Analyzing
Client Need: Physiological Integrity

5 - 3

① **The younger the child, the greater the volume of fluid needed in proportion to body weight. At 6 years of age, the client's body surface in proportion to body weight leads to increased insensible fluid loss through the skin.**

2. The proportion of body weight contributed by water is greater, not smaller, during early childhood compared to adulthood.

3. The kidneys are functionally mature at birth.

4. The total volume of extracellular fluid per kilogram of body weight does not increase gradually from birth to adolescence. As a person matures, body fluid will decrease due to body growth.

Nursing Process: Analyzing
Client Need: Health Promotion and Maintenance

5 - 4

① **In this situation, the nurse should wash hands, don clean gloves, remove soiled dressing, wash hands, prepare sterile field, and don sterile gloves. Nurses should wash their hands first before beginning any procedure.**

2, 3, and 4. None of these options follow the required sequence necessary to maintain sterile technique.

Nursing Process: Implementing
Client Need: Safe, Effective Care Environment

5 - 5

② **Keeping an infant's fingernails cut short will lessen the chance of secondary infection and the "itch-scratch-itch" cycle. Infants with atopic dermatitis (eczema) may try to scratch themselves because of intense itching.**

1. Soaps should be avoided because of the drying effects they have on the skin. Dry skin triggers and exacerbates atopic dermatitis.

3. Long-sleeved clothing is recommended because it discourages scratching. Also, it is advisable to wear soft cotton fabrics next to the skin.

4. Atopic dermatitis is not contagious. There is no need for family members to avoid a child with this condition.

Nursing Process: Implementing
Client Need: Health Promotion and Maintenance

5 - 6

④ **Benzoyl peroxide is an anti-acne medication whose action is due to its bacteriostatic properties and its penetration. Acne vulgaris is a common skin disorder of adolescents that is caused by the microorganism *P. acnes.***

1, 2, and 3. Amphotericin B, ciclopirox olamine (Loprox), and butoconazole nitrate (Femstat) are all antifungal agents and do not have an impact on acne vulgaris.

Nursing Process: Assessing
Client Need: Health Promotion and Maintenance

5 - 7

③ **The nurse will remove all clothing and cover the client in a clean sheet. The initial treatment of a burn victim includes removing clothing and covering the victim. Clothing may still be smoldering and may increase the extent of the burn. Also, a complete assessment must be done. In this instance, it is very probable that the burns, which involve all layers of the skin, are painless. Severe painless burns are often the most serious because even the nerve endings have been damaged.**

1 and 2. In order to allow a thorough survey and assessment and to avoid further injury due to smoldering garments, clothing of the burn victim should be removed.

4. Oil-based ointments are contraindicated in the initial treatment of burns. The initial application to burned skin is usually a cooling liquid such as chilled saline or water.

Nursing Process: Implementing
Client Need: Safe, Effective Care Environment

5 - 8

② **Morphine sulfate (Morphine) is an opioid analgesic whose impact on the central nervous system makes it a very potent pain reliever. Because of the very painful nature of second-degree burns, adequate pain management is a challenge and is likely to necessitate an opioid.**

1 and 3. Acetaminophen (Tylenol) and ibuprofen (Motrin) are used to treat mild to moderate pain.

4. A transcutaneous electrical nerve stimulation (TENS) unit is for localized pain and is attached to the skin, making it unsuitable for burn analgesia.

Nursing Process: Planning
Client Need: Physiological Integrity

5 - 9

④ **Tetanus prophylaxis is indicated for any client who has a nonsurgical wound or injury and has not received a tetanus immunization within 10 years. Unlike some other diseases that are considered eradicated, such as smallpox, tetanus remains a threat to people who are not immunized and have a break in their skin's integrity. Only those allergic to the injection are exempt.**

1. Casting is not an acceptable treatment for deep partial-thickness burns. These injuries require dressings.

2. Fungal infections are much less common in the burn injury than bacterial infections, so bacteriostatic ointments are used to prevent infection.

3. Surgical intervention is usually not required in deep partial-thickness burns. All full-thickness burns require surgical consultation at least.

Nursing Process: Planning
Client Need: Physiological Integrity

5 - 1 0

④ **The chief purpose for hydrotherapy for clients with extensive burns is to cleanse the wounds by removing loose tissue and debris. Hydrotherapy also allows for active range-of-motion exercises.**

1. The prevention of infection is accomplished by use of topical silver sulfadiazine (Silvadene).
2. Fluid replacement is essential and is achieved through intravenous infusion (IV). Burn shock requires IV administration of fluid to maintain circulating volume.
3. Wounds are not sterile; therefore, using an antibacterial soap is not necessary.

Nursing Process: Implementing
Client Need: Physiological Integrity

5 - 1 1

④ **To keep the donor site soft and scarring at a minimum, lotion or lanolin cream should be applied several times a day.**

1, 2, and 3. Soaps and hydrogen peroxide are irritants and should be avoided.

Nursing Process: Implementing
Client Need: Health Promotion and Maintenance

5 - 1 2

③ **Temperature reduction is promoted by the evaporation of moisture from the skin. This is the desired outcome of the procedure.**

1. Friction produces heat and would be counterproductive.
2. Offering fluids would affect hydration but would not directly affect body temperature.
4. Lowering room temperature could cause chilling and sudden fluctuations in the client's body temperature.

Nursing Process: Implementing
Client Need: Safe, Effective Care Environment

5 - 13

① Rifampin (Rifadin) and dapsone (Avlosulfont) are antitubercular antileprotics that are used as first-line pharmacologic treatment on skin and mucosal lesions such as those associated with Hansen's disease (leprosy).

2. Amphotericin B (Fungizone) and nystatin (Mycostatin) are antifungal agents administered to treat fungal infections. They do not have an impact on bacteria.

3. Cicloprirox (Loprox) and haloprogin (Halotex) are antifungal agents and do not impact on bacteria.

4. Miconazole (Monistat) and clotrimazole (Mycelex G) are antifungal agents and do not impact on bacteria.

Nursing Process: Assessing

Client Need: Physiological Integrity

5 - 14

③ Meperidine (Demerol) would be appropriate to administer one-half hour prior to the debridement of a full-thickness burn. Demerol is an opioid analgesic whose effect on pain perception makes it a very effective analgesic. Because of the painful nature of many burn debridements, analgesia is often given beforehand.

1. Acetaminophen (Tylenol) is an antipyretic analgesic indicated for mild or moderate pain only.

2. Fluoxetine (Prozac) is an antidepressant medication.

4. Captopril (Capoten) is an antihypertensive medication.

Nursing Process: Implementing

Client Need: Health Promotion and Maintenance

5 - 1 5

④ **The nurse would prepare lactated Ringer's (LR) solution. There are numerous formulas used to calculate intravenous replacement for burn victims. The consensus formula is simply:**

$$\frac{2 \text{ to } 4 \text{ ml} \times \text{kg body weight} \times \% \text{ body surface area burned}}{2}$$

If the average adult weighs approximately 75 kg, one might quickly estimate:

$$\frac{3 \text{ ml} \times 75 \text{ kg} \times 18\%}{2} = 2,025 \text{ in 8 hours or 250 cc LR per hr.}$$

1. Normal saline at a keep-vein-open (KVO) rate is too slow to rehydrate a burned client.
2. Lidocaine (20 to 50 mg/kg per min) infusion is administered to treat ventricular arrhythmias, not to rehydrate clients who have been burned.
3. Dextrose 5% in water (D5W) administered at a keep-vein-open (KVO) rate is too slow to rehydrate a burned client.

Nursing Process: Planning

Client Need: Physiological Integrity

5 - 1 6

③ **A large amount of blood-tinged, drainage is expected and the dressing should be reinforced. It is the purpose of a wound drain to prevent the accumulation of blood in the wound.**

1. Since the drainage is blood-tinged, it cannot be hemorrhage. Venous blood is dark and arterial blood is bright red.
2. There is no indication that a dehiscence (bursting open of a wound) is imminent.
4. There is no indication that the wound is obstructed. In fact, the dressing is saturated with blood-tinged drainage.

Nursing Process: Analyzing

Client Need: Health Promotion and Maintenance

5 - 1 7

③ **The nurse should turn and reposition the client. Turning and repositioning the client every 1 to 2 hours will relieve pressure and aid in the prevention of skin breakdown.**

1. Coughing and deep breathing will help to prevent pneumonia and atelectasis, not pressure ulcers.
2. Massaging the extremities is not recommended since edema interferes with circulation and the development of thrombi is possible.
4. Lamb's wool would be helpful, but not as effective as repositioning the client every 1 to 2 hours.

Nursing Process: Implementing

Client Need: Health Promotion and Maintenance

5 - 1 8

① **Arterial blood gases (ABGs) should be drawn. Arterial blood gases are usually the first laboratory evaluation performed on clients who have been burned in order to establish pulmonary function levels.**

2. Although pain relief is an important consideration, intramuscular medications are not indicated. Intravenous medications are not administered until fluid resuscitation is completed.

3. Assessment of the client's home environment is a lower-level priority in the immediate care of clients who are burned.

4. Body weight assessments are useful to determine fluid resuscitation requirements, but this does not take priority over pulmonary function levels that may indicate airway obstruction.

Nursing Process: Assessing
Client Need: Physiological Integrity

5 - 1 9

① **The client has probably sustained a superficial partial-thickness burn. Superficial partial-thickness burns are usually very painful, have hair follicles present, are intact, and will usually heal on their own if they are not complicated by infection. A prolonged exposure to the sun's rays can cause a superficial partial-thickness burn, which is typically called a "sunburn". All clients should be advised to wear protective clothing or sunscreen to protect against such an injury.**

2. Deep partial-thickness burns are less common in the sun-exposed client who is conscious and able to retreat from the sun's rays.

3. Full-thickness burns, which involve all layers of the skin, are usually caused by hot liquids or fire.

4. Sunburn is a very real injury and should be treated as such.

Nursing Process: Implementing
Client Need: Physiological Integrity

5-20

③ **Edema is the first consequence of capillary permeability in the surrounding tissue of clients who are burned. Increased capillary permeability is a direct cause of edema. As the capillary walls become more permeable, water, sodium, and other proteins such as albumin move into the interstitial spaces surrounding the affected tissue.**

1. Body fluid loss occurs as a consequence of edema.

2. Pain is not the first consequence of increased capillary permeability. Pain develops as a consequence of edema pressing against the nerve endings.

4. Nausea is often associated with intense feelings of pain and is not the first consequence of increased capillary permeability.

Nursing Process: Assessing

Client Need: Physiological Integrity

5-21

① **The lowest priority data to collect at this time would be body weight. Body weight is obtained initially to help calculate drug dosage and fluid requirements. There will be little change of body weight in 24 hours.**

2. A partial paralytic ileus may occur in children with 20% or greater burns, most often in the first 2 to 3 days. Therefore, bowel sounds should be assessed.

3. Breath sounds should be assessed since common pulmonary problems include infections, aspiration, inhalation, and pulmonary edema.

4. Vital signs can give data about fluid status and infection and should be assessed often.

Nursing Process: Evaluating

Client Need: Physiological Integrity

5-22

② **Eighteen percent of a client's body is affected if the anterior chest and abdomen are burned. The "rule of nines" is a quick assessment used to evaluate the extent of a victim's burn injury based on body surface. It does not address the thickness of the injury. Using the "rule of nines", an adult's head and neck are assigned 9% of the body surface, the upper right extremity 9%, the upper left extremity 9%, the anterior chest and abdomen 18%, the posterior chest and abdomen 18%, each leg 18%, and the perineal area 1%. Treatment is based on the extent and depth of injuries.**

1, 3, and 4. All are incorrect calculations using the "rule of nines."

Nursing Process: Assessing

Client Need: Physiological Integrity

5-23

① The nurse can reduce sources of heat from a client's body by removing metals such as jewelry, coins, eyeglasses, and watches. Metals retain heat once exposed to fire.

2, 3, and 4. Dentures, makeup, and hairpieces should be removed to facilitate assessment of the client. However, these articles do not retain heat like metals.

Nursing Process: Implementing
Client Need: Physiological Integrity

5-24

② Clients with fungal skin infections should avoid the use of cornstarch. Fungal or mycotic skin infections may be due to numerous microorganisms. These infections are nourished by non-human nutrients. The carbohydrates in cornstarch may provide nutrition to fungal infection and should be avoided.

1 and 3. There is no evidence that detergents or cotton clothing will worsen a fungal infection.

4. There are many effective antifungal creams available, such as nystatin (Mycostatin) and oxiconazole nitrate (Oxistat).

Nursing Process: Implementing
Client Need: Safe, Effective Care Environment

5-25

④ The client should be taught to taper the dosage of prednisone. Prednisone, like all glucocorticoids, is normally produced by the adrenal glands. Exogenous replacement of this hormone will interrupt the adrenal's normal hormone production. Abrupt cessation may cause adrenal crisis.

1. Prednisone should be taken on schedule, not as needed (prn).

2. There is no indication that prednisone must be taken with orange juice.

3. The physician should prescribe any needed medication for future illness.

Nursing Process: Implementing
Client Need: Health Promotion and Maintenance

5-26

① Tetracycline (Tetracap) is an antibacterial agent that may be taken orally to treat severe cases of acne, or it may be applied topically as a cream. Acne is a common skin disorder of adolescence and is caused by the bacterium *P. acnes*.

2. Pyrimethamine (Daraprim) is an antimalarial agent and does not have an impact on bacterial infections.

3. Miconazole (Monistat) is an antifungal agent and does not have an impact on bacterial infections.

4. Famciclovir (Famvir) is an antiviral agent and does not have an impact on bacterial infections.

Nursing Process: Implementing

Client Need: Health Promotion and Maintenance

5-27

② You will teach clients with anemia that pruritus occurs as a result of increased serum and skin bile salt concentrations.

1. The pallor seen in clients with anemia is a result of reduced hemoglobin and decreased blood flow to the skin.

3. The jaundice seen in clients with anemia is a result of increased concentration of serum bilirubin that increases red blood cell hemolysis.

4. Low viscosity of blood occurs in clients with severe anemia. It does not affect the integumentary system, but it may contribute to systolic murmurs.

Nursing Process: Implementing

Client Need: Physiological Integrity

5-28

④ The nurse should advise parents to avoid applying diphenhydramine (Benadryl) liberally over the entire body of their child. Diphenhydramine affects the inflammatory response. It is an antihistamine that is very useful in relieving local skin irritation when applied topically. It is, however, absorbed systemically, especially if open lesions are present. Dosing may be excessive if ointment is applied too liberally.

1. Calamine lotion is a drying agent and would be an appropriate treatment.

2. Acetaminophen (Tylenol) is an analgesic antipyretic and would be an appropriate treatment.

3. Diphenhydramine is an antihistamine that can provide relief from the discomfort of chicken pox when taken po as directed.

Nursing Process: Planning

Client Need: Physiological Integrity

5 - 2 9

① A partial-thickness (first-degree) burn only affects the epidermis. With a first-degree burn, pain and mild edema occur. However, there are no blisters. An example of a first-degree burn would be a superficial sunburn.

2. Deep (second-degree) burns involve the epidermis and dermis. Vesicles develop and clients experience severe pain caused by nerve injury.

3 and 4. Full-thickness burns involve the epidermis, dermis, subcutaneous tissue, and destruction of nerve endings. Coagulation necrosis is also present.

Nursing Process: Assessing
Client Need: Physiological Integrity

5 - 3 0

③ You will teach the caregiver of a child with cellulitis how to apply warm, moist compresses to the affected area. Cellulitis is a bacterial infection caused by streptococcus. Treatment includes oral antibiotics such as penicillin and erythromycin. Warm, moist soaks are applied every 4 hours to increase circulation and relieve pain.

1 and 2. The use of elastic pressure bandages and elbow restraints will compromise circulation and are contraindicated.

4. Movement is not encouraged. The child should rest in bed with the affected arm elevated and immobilized.

Nursing Process: Implementing
Client Need: Physiological Integrity

5 - 3 1

① The nurse will inform the client that the medication podofilox (Condylox) is contraindicated during pregnancy because of its abortifacient properties (causes or induces abortion). Podofilox places the developing fetus at risk because of its potentially myelotoxic (destructive to bone marrow) and neurotoxic (destructive to nerve cells) properties. Condylomata acuminata (genital warts) are caused by a virus and cannot be cured because there is no specific antiviral therapy.

2. Podofilox is available only in a 0.5% topical solution.

3. Podofilox is contraindicated during pregnancy because of its abortifacient properties.

4. The client should not continue to treat the condition with this medication. Other treatments include cryotherapy using liquid oxygen, cryoprobe, carbon dioxide lasers, electrocautery, and surgical incision.

Nursing Process: Implementing
Client Need: Health Promotion and Maintenance

5 - 3 2

④ **The nurse will teach parents not to cover areas of their child's skin affected by impetigo. Areas of the skin affected by impetigo should be left open to the air. Impetigo is the most common childhood infection of the skin. It is caused by staphylococcus aureus. The lesions can be spread simply by touching an unaffected part of the skin after scratching an infected area. Thorough and frequent hand washing cannot be overemphasized on the part of the child and parents.**

1. Treatment of impetigo includes washing and soaking the lesion 3 times a day in warm soapy water.

2. Crusts should be removed after soaking.

3. Applying topical antibiotic ointment and leaving the areas open to the air are appropriate interventions.

Nursing Process: Implementing

Client Need: Physiological Integrity

5 - 3 3

④ **The nurse will teach the parents that only one application of permethrin 1% (Nix) is necessary since it kills both lice and eggs (pediculosis capitis).**

1. Applying the medication after the hair is shampooed, rinsed, and dried is the correct procedure.

2. Between 25 to 50 ml of the liquid medication is recommended to saturate the hair and scalp.

3. It is recommended that the medication remain on the hair and scalp for 10 minutes before rinsing off with water.

Nursing Process: Implementing

Client Need: Health Promotion and Maintenance

5 - 3 4

③ **Vitiligo is best described as unpigmented skin patches associated with lack of melanin formation. The condition is more common among black clients.**

1. Keloids are raised, firm, thickened, red scars that form at the site of a wound. The abnormal increase in scar size is due to unusually high amounts of collagen deposits in the tissue.

2. Pseudofolliculitis ("razor bumps") are so-called ingrown hairs that produce symptoms that include papules, pustules, and keloids.

4. Tinea versicolor is a fungal infection that produces yellow- or fawn-colored patches on the skin.

Nursing Process: Assessing

Client Need: Physiological Integrity

5-35

② **The least likely plan of care would include the use of hydrotherapy to stimulate circulation. Clients with autografts should not be immersed or showered until the graft has taken and the wound is closed.**

1. The supine position (lying on the back with face upward) will allow the graft to remain in place.
3. Elbow restraints are required to keep the child's hands away from the affected area.
4. Aspiration of fluid accumulation under the graft will help the graft to remain flat and in full contact with the tissue bed below.

Nursing Process: Planning
Client Need: Physiological Integrity

5-36

① **Nursing assessment will reveal restlessness in the early stages of shock. Other assessment findings include increase in blood pressure, deeper respirations, and a slight decrease in urinary output. These findings, however, are within normal limits. Shock is circulatory failure resulting in impaired tissue perfusion that leads to cellular dysfunction.**

2. There will be a marked increase in blood pressure, not a decrease.
3. The respirations will not be shallow but progressively deeper.
4. The client's urinary output will have a slight decrease but not to the extent of oliguria.

Nursing Process: Assessing
Client Need: Physiological Integrity

5-37

③ **The most appropriate nursing diagnosis for a neonate under a radiant warmer receiving phototherapy is: fluid volume deficit, potential for.**

1. There should be no problems with the neonate's skin integrity if the neonate is turned every 2 hours.
2. There is no association between gas exchange and the use of a radiant warmer.
4. There is no association between infection and the use of a radiant warmer.

Nursing Process: Assessing
Client Need: Physiological Integrity

5 - 3 8

③ **Aseptic technique reduces the risk of introducing additional microorganisms into the wound.**

1 and 2. Warm, moist packs are not bactericidal. An anti-infective might be prescribed to kill or inhibit the growth of pathogenic bacteria.

4. To minimize the risk of spreading infection to others, the nurse would dispose of all contaminated materials properly.

Nursing Process: Implementing
Client Need: Safe, Effective Care Environment

5 - 3 9

① **Mongolian spotting (blue-gray pigmentation) over the buttocks and sacrum is not associated with congenital anomalies. The spotting occurs most often in dark-skinned clients and disappears on its own during early childhood.**

2. Short stature, low posterior hairline, webbing of neck, broad chest, and widely spaced nipples are physical characteristics of an infant born with Turner's syndrome (45,XO).

3. A simian crease across the palms of both hands is associated with trisomy 21 (Down syndrome).

4. Low ears are associated with a number of congenital anomalies such as Down syndrome (trisomy 21) and Edward's syndrome (trisomy 18).

Nursing Process: Assessing
Client Need: Physiological Integrity

5 - 4 0

② **A dark-skinned client's skin will appear dusky red or violet with erythema (a form of macula). A light-skinned client's skin will appear diffusely red.**

1. Paleness is loss of skin color. For example, clients with anemia may experience paleness.

3. Dark-skinned clients experiencing cyanosis will appear black while light-skinned clients experiencing cyanosis appear blue or dark purple.

4. A temporary yellow discoloration of the skin of light-skinned clients may indicate jaundice. A dark-skinned client with jaundice would manifest the condition by a yellow appearance in the sclera of the eyes, mucous membranes, and body fluids.

Nursing Process: Assessing
Client Need: Physiological Integrity

Practice Test 6

Musculoskeletal System

6 - 1

A child is in a hip spica cast. Discharge instruction should include teaching the parents to move the child from room to room to change diversions frequently. This is most important for a child in which age group?

1. toddlers
2. preschoolers
3. school-age children
4. adolescents

6 - 2

Your client has been scheduled for an arthroscopy following an injury to the left knee. After the arthroscopy, the joint will be wrapped with a compress dressing and the affected leg will be:

1. placed in a flexed position by placing a pillow under the knee.
2. kept in an extended position and elevated.
3. placed in a slightly flexed position and elevated.
4. placed flat on the bed with a trochanter roll on either side of the knee.

6 - 3

Your client is scheduled for an electromyography today. What do you need to do to prepare your client for this procedure?

1. Maintain nothing by mouth for 6 hours prior to the procedure.
2. Omit any scheduled diazepam for 24 hours prior to the procedure.
3. Inform the client that he will not feel any pain during the procedure.
4. Inform the client that he will have to lie still during the procedure.

6 - 4

An infant is being treated for congenital hip dysplasia with a Pavlik harness. Teaching about care of the infant has been effective if the caregiver:

1. maintains the infant's leg position with a smaller pillow or foam wedge during diaper change.
2. carefully inspects and cleans the inguinal area during a diaper change.
3. places an undershirt over the harness to minimize soiling.
4. releases the straps 4 times a day 1 at a time and inspects the skin underneath.

6 - 5

An infant is being treated for bilateral club-foot with long leg casts. Treatment began at 2 weeks of age and will continue for 3 months. Education about home care should include:

1. keeping the child's hands diverted so that objects won't be inserted under the cast.
2. outlining areas of blood on the cast and noting the time.
3. handling the casts with fingertips, not palms of hands
4. checking circulation in the toes frequently, at least with each diaper change.

6 - 6

An 84-year-old client asks the nurse, "Why am I 5'3" now, but was 5'7" when I graduated from high school?" The nurse's best response would be to say:

1. "I will be glad to measure your height now and see how tall you really are."
2. "Whoever measured your height last must have made a mistake since you know you were 5'7" in high school."
3. "It's possible you weren't standing as straight as you could have been when your height was measured."
4. "The disks in your backbone have become thinner as you have gotten older."

6 - 7

An athlete fell and broke the radius in the right arm. Following the application of a cast, the athlete says to you, "I'm afraid I'm going to lose muscle strength in my arm because I can't exercise it." Your best response would be:

1. "It must be difficult for an athlete to be unable to maintain an exercise program because of injuries."
2. "You can minimize the effects of immobility by performing isometric exercises of the immobilized muscles."
3. "Would you like for me to speak with the physician about participating in a physical therapy program?"
4. "There will be some atrophy of the muscle. However, you should be able to regain full muscle strength once the cast is removed."

6 - 8

A client is suspected of having metastatic bone disease. To aid in the confirmation of this condition, you anticipate which of the following?

1. venogram
2. discography
3. electromyography
4. bone scan

6 - 9

A fracture of your client's acetabulum is suspected. Which of the following diagnostic tools is most likely to be used to identify the specific location and extent of the suspected injury?

1. angiography
2. magnetic resonance imaging
3. computed tomography
4. arthroscopy

6 - 10

During the assessment of a 76-year-old client, you notice an increased roundness of the thoracic spinal curve. You will document this observation as:

1. scoliosis.
2. osteoporosis.
3. kyphosis.
4. lordosis.

6 - 11

Your client experienced a fractured ulna. You observe swelling at the site of injury and the client is complaining of pain. The client is in which stage of bone healing?

1. inflammatory
2. cellular proliferation
3. callus formation
4. ossification

6 - 1 2

A client was admitted to your unit with carpal tunnel syndrome. What will you expect your assessment to reveal?

1. weakened grasp
2. shoulder pain in the deltoid area
3. flexion of the fourth and fifth fingers
4. numbness of the thumb and first and second fingers

6 - 1 3

The nurse in the newborn nursery has completed an initial physical assessment. Observations reveal asymmetry of gluteal folds with a positive Ortolani's sign. The most likely implication of this finding would be:

1. congenital hip dysplasia.
2. normal examination of the hip.
3. cerebral palsy.
4. rickets.

6 - 1 4

Your 76-year-old client has developed contractures. In order to prevent the contractures from becoming worse, you will:

1. place the client in a warm whirlpool bath daily.
2. perform range-of-motion exercises qid.
3. turn the client from side to side every 2 hours.
4. support contracted joints on pillows at all times.

6 - 1 5

A client has sustained a closed fracture of the humerus. After application of the cast, the nurse teaches the client about cast care. Which of the following measures would be contraindicated?

1. Avoid putting powder around the cast edges.
2. Place a plastic bag over the cast while bathing.
3. Call the physician if drainage or odors are observed around the cast.
4. Use a coat hanger to relieve itching under the cast.

6 - 1 6

A client was admitted to the nursing unit with soft tissue injury following a snakebite on the right index finger. The client's fingers are cold and pale on the affected hand. What should the nurse do first?

1. Elevate the extremity.
2. Administer pain medication.
3. Call the physician.
4. Provide passive range-of-motion exercises to the client's fingers.

6 - 1 7

A 12-year-old in a spica cast complains of discomfort after eating. Which of the following measures should the nurse take to prevent this problem?

1. Give the client smaller but more frequent meals.
2. Continue to give the client 3 meals a day, but give smaller portions.
3. Restrict the fluid intake.
4. Encourage the client to eat slowly and to alternate liquids with solids.

6 - 1 8

Your client had a bilateral total knee replacement to treat degenerative joint disease. During the first 24 to 72 hours after surgery, you will assess for which of the following?

1. bowel impaction and abdominal pain
2. confusion, dyspnea, and petechiae
3. redness and edema at the incision site
4. pedal pulses

6 - 1 9

What type of gait would be utilized by a client with a broken leg who is walking up stairs with the assistance of crutches?

1. 2-point
2. modified 3-point
3. 4-point
4. swing-through

6-20

A client is experiencing weakness in the left leg and is learning to use a walker. Which observation made by the nurse would indicate that the client understands the instructions given?

1. The client advances the walker and steps forward, alternating the feet with each advancement.
2. The client advances both feet, moves the walker forward, then moves both feet again.
3. The client advances the walker and steps forward with the left foot at the same time.
4. The client advances the right foot and then moves the walker forward, dragging the left foot.

6-21

Which statement is correct concerning the best method of performing passive range-of-motion exercises?

1. A joint should never be forced beyond its capacity.
2. Range-of-motion exercises will cause some discomfort if they are to be beneficial.
3. Support should be maintained above the joint being exercised.
4. Range-of-motion movements should be repeated a minimum of 10 times.

6-22

A client is to have a modified radical mastectomy. While the nurse is giving instructions on arm exercises prior to surgery, the client asks, "Why will I have to exercise my arm after surgery, when it will hurt?" Which of the following responses would be best for the nurse to make?

1. "These exercises prevent stiffness of the shoulder and help you regain use of your arm."
2. "Exercising the arm will actually decrease the amount of postoperative pain."
3. "Exercises will eliminate the postoperative swelling that occurs at the incision."
4. "You are practicing now so that it won't be so uncomfortable for you later."

6 - 2 3

Which of the following assessment observations indicates scoliosis?

1. head in alignment with gluteal fold
2. symmetrical thoracic area
3. equal leg length
4. asymmetry in the flank area

6 - 2 4

An adult client has experienced a bone marrow aspiration. Immediately following this procedure, the nurse will:

1. apply firm pressure to the site of the aspiration for at least 5 minutes.
2. place a plain adhesive bandage over the aspiration site.
3. apply a topical antibiotic on the aspiration site and leave open.
4. apply an ice pack to the aspiration site for at least 10 minutes.

6 - 2 5

An 11-month-old infant has been placed in Bryant's traction for treatment of a fractured femur. The plan of care will include:

1. turning the child from side to side at least every 2 hours.
2. elevating the head of the bed 15 to 30 degrees when meals are served.
3. keeping pin insertion sites clean and free from exudate.
4. keeping toys within easy reach of the child.

6 - 2 6

Your client is in traction to treat a fractured femur. The physician has prescribed a 2-view X ray of the femur. Which of the following is contraindicated as a nursing action?

1. Release the weight of the traction to move the client to the radiology department.
2. Maintain the correct body alignment while positioning for the X ray.
3. Administer pain medication 30 minutes following the procedure.
4. Explain the procedure to the client.

6 - 2 7

When assisting clients with walkers, it would be best for the nurse to walk:

1. directly behind the client.
2. in front of the client, guiding the walker.
3. closely behind and slightly to the side of the client.
4. beside the client.

6 - 2 8

Following a simple mandibular fracture, your client is scheduled for an intermaxillary fixation. Immediately after surgery, you will place the client in which position?

1. a side-lying position with the head slightly elevated
2. an upright position with the neck flexed
3. a horizontal recumbent position
4. a prone position

6 - 2 9

Which of the following self-care behaviors should the nurse include when teaching a client about a continuous passive motion machine?

1. how to operate the on/off switch
2. how to increase/decrease flexion and extension movements
3. how to adjust speed controls
4. how to adjust internal and external rotation movements

6 - 3 0

A 7-year-old child has juvenile rheumatoid arthritis. During a period of exacerbation, the plan of care will include:

1. clustering of care to allow uninterrupted periods of rest.
2. short-term use of narcotics administered by client-controlled analgesia.
3. a high-protein, high-vitamin diet.
4. cool packs to the inflamed joints bid and hs.

6 - 3 1

A client fractured his left femur during a soccer game. During your initial assessment in the Emergency Department, the client says, "My leg feels numb." You understand that the probable cause of the numbness is:

1. blood loss.
2. nerve damage.
3. paralysis.
4. muscle spasms.

6 - 3 2

Your client has had a total hip replacement and you are changing the client's position. Which action should you take to prevent hip dislocation?

1. Cross the client's legs at the knees.
2. Place a pillow along the client's back.
3. Use a drawsheet to facilitate turning the client.
4. Support the client's legs with abductor pillow between the legs.

6 - 3 3

Which of the following medications might contribute to the further development of osteoporosis?

1. methylprednisolone 8 mg po, qid
2. calcium carbonate 500 mg po, qid
3. ranitidine 150 mg po, bid
4. ramipril 10 mg po, qid

6 - 3 4

A 67-year-old client comes to the local clinic with acute gouty arthritis. An immediate nursing intervention would be to:

1. relieve pain.
2. administer anti-inflammatory agents.
3. relieve pressure on the tender joints.
4. apply cold packs to reduce inflammation.

6 - 3 5

A client complains of feeling faint following a traumatic fracture. The nurse's assessment reveals dyspnea, restlessness, tachycardia, progressive cyanosis, and mental confusion. Which of the following complications will the nurse suspect?

1. nerve damage
2. fat embolism
3. hypostatic pneumonia
4. progressing paralysis

6 - 3 6

A client is experiencing left-sided weakness. You are to get the client into a wheelchair. The intravenous pole and nasogastric suction equipment are on the left side of the bed. Where should you position the wheelchair prior to transfer?

1. on the left side of the bed with the wheelchair facing the head of the bed
2. on the right side of the bed with the wheelchair facing the head of the bed
3. on the left side of the bed with the wheelchair facing the foot of the bed
4. on the right side of the bed with the wheelchair facing the foot of the bed

6 - 3 7

A 9-year-old has a fractured left femur and a long leg cast has been applied. Which of the following behaviors by the client indicates acceptance of the cast?

1. The client whittles at the cast with a table knife.
2. The client asks for help to replace the waterproof petal around the edges of the cast.
3. The client stuffs paper inside the cast.
4. The client refuses to go to the playroom.

6 - 3 8

Which of the following crutch gaits would be appropriate for a client with paralysis of the legs and hips?

1. the 4-point gait
2. the 3-point gait
3. the swing-through gait
4. the 2-point gait

6 - 3 9

An 8-year-old client fractured the right femur and is in 90-90 traction. Three of the following options describe purposes of traction. Which of the following is not a purpose of traction?

1. to reduce dislocation
2. to immobilize the leg
3. to lessen muscle spasm
4. to provide comfort

6 - 4 0

Which of the following is the appropriate site for an intramuscular injection for an infant 6 months of age?

1. deltoid
2. vastus lateralis
3. dorsogluteal
4. ventrogluteal

6 - 4 1

In addition to local joint symptoms, which of the following manifestations are common in clients who have rheumatoid arthritis?

1. pedal edema
2. generalized erythema
3. fever and complaints of fatigue
4. bradycardia and slow respirations

6 - 4 2

Management for a client who has sustained a musculoskeletal injury due to dislocation will require immediate intervention. The need for immediate intervention is based on the possible development of:

1. shock.
2. inadequate blood supply.
3. fat embolism.
4. contractures.

6 - 4 3

A client had the right leg amputated above the knee as the result of an automobile accident. Immediately following the surgery, the nurse will know to place the client's affected limb in a position of:

1. extension.
2. flexion.
3. internal rotation.
4. external rotation.

6 - 4 4

A 45-year-old is suspected of having myasthenia gravis. To confirm this tentative diagnosis, the nurse will anticipate a prescription for which of the following diagnostic tests?

1. tensilon test
2. cold stimulation test
3. magnetic resonance imaging
4. electroencephalography

Practice Test 6

Answers, Rationales, and Explanations

6 - 1

① Toddlers are involved in environmental exploration, especially through use of large muscles. Confinement can hinder autonomy and speech development. Toddlers also have a short attention span.

2, 3, and 4. Preschoolers, school-age children, and adolescents have a longer attention span and greater capacity for self-direction.

Nursing Process: Implementing
Client Need: Psychosocial Integrity

6 - 2

② Immediately following an arthroscopy of the knee, the nurse will elevate the leg with the knee in an extended position. This will reduce swelling and pain. An arthroscopy is an endoscopic procedure that allows for direct visualization of joints.

1 and 3. The affected joint should be extended, not flexed, following an arthroscopy. Extension will prevent edema and take pressure off the joint.

4. The leg should be elevated to help prevent edema.

Nursing Process: Implementing
Client Need: Health Promotion and Maintenance

6 - 3

② Persons scheduled for electromyography (EMG) should omit diazepam (Valium) since it causes loss of muscle tonicity. Electromyography aids in the diagnosis of muscular dystrophy, amyotrophic lateral sclerosis, and myasthenia gravis by evaluating electrical potential associated with skeletal muscle contraction. Clients may have to move their muscles voluntarily during the procedure and they may experience some discomfort from needle insertion.

1. There is no special client preparation required prior to an electromyography.

3. The client should be told that a sensation similar to receiving an intramuscular injection will be experienced and that the muscle may ache for a short period of time afterward.

4. Because the client may need to move muscles voluntarily, it is not necessary that they lie still during the procedure.

Nursing Process: Planning
Client Need: Psychosocial Integrity

6 - 4

② **The nurse will know that teaching has been effective if the caregiver carefully inspects and cleans the inguinal area during a diaper change. The skin surfaces of the inguinal area are especially prone to breakdown because of thigh flexion.**

1. The caregiver should be taught that the harness will maintain positioning during diaper change.
3. To help prevent skin irritation, the infant's undershirt should be placed under the harness.
4. The harness should be removed only for bathing or not at all according to the prescription.

Nursing Process: Implementing

Client Need: Health Promotion and Maintenance

6 - 5

④ **An infant being treated for bilateral clubfoot with long leg casts should have circulation checks of the toes with each diaper change. Even though casts are changed often (every few days for 1 to 2 weeks, then at 1- to 2-week intervals), the child will be growing rapidly and could develop circulatory impairment.**

1. An infant is not likely to be capable of stuffing objects under the cast.
2. Casting does not require surgery. Therefore, bleeding is not a concern.
3. Handling hardening casts should be done with palms of hands, not fingertips. Fingertips tend to press into the cast and create pressure areas that could compromise skin integrity.

Nursing Process: Implementing

Client Need: Physiological Integrity

6 - 6

④ **The client should be taught that thinning of the intervertebral disks occurs with age. Other gerontologic changes may include weakened muscles, osteoporotic bones, enlarged joints, and decreased range of motion. The nurse will also teach the client how to minimize the effects of aging.**

1. Offering to measure the client's height suggests some error has been made. It is likely that no error was made and that the client has lost 4 inches of height due to intervertebral thinning.
2. No error was made. The client has lost 4 inches of height due to thinning of the intervertebral disks.
3. The nurse should not attempt to pacify the client by suggesting that the client was not standing erect at the time of the last height measurement. The client should be told about various changes that occur during the aging process and how to minimize their effects.

Nursing Process: Implementing

Client Need: Health Promotion and Maintenance

6 - 7

② **Clients who are concerned about loss of muscle strength due to casting should be taught that they can minimize the loss by performing isometric exercises. Isometric exercises may be defined as contraction of a muscle that is not accompanied by motion of the joints that would ordinarily be moved by that contraction.**

1. Telling the client that it must be difficult to be unable to exercise because of an injury leaves the client with the impression there is nothing that can be done to minimize muscle loss until the cast is removed. The client could perform isometric exercises on the affected arm.

3. The physical therapy department may be contacted. However, the nurse should encourage the client by teaching the client about the therapeutic benefits of isometric exercises.

4. The client needs to know that isometric exercises can be performed while the affected arm is in a cast.

Nursing Process: Implementing
Client Need: Physiological Integrity

6 - 8

④ **A bone scan (bone scintigraphy) would be anticipated to aid in the confirmation of suspected metastatic bone disease. Radioactive isotopes search out bone. The degree of isotope uptake by the bone indicates the presence of conditions such as osteosarcoma, metastatic bone disease, and osteomyelitis.**

1. Venograms are used to study the venous system and help to identify conditions such as venous thrombosis. A venogram would not detect bony metastasis.

2. Discography is a test to study intervertebral discs, requiring a contrast medium that is injected into the discs. A discography would not detect bony metastasis.

3. Electromyography is a diagnostic tool that provides information about the electrical condition of the muscles and the nerves leading to muscles. An electromyography would not detect bony metastasis.

Nursing Process: Planning
Client Need: Physiological Integrity

6 - 9

③ **The nurse will anticipate a prescription for computed tomography (CT scan). The CT scan is very useful in identifying soft tissue injuries to ligaments and tendons. Also, the presence of tumors can be identified and the extent and location of fractures in areas that are hard to evaluate, such as the acetabulum (the rounded cavity that holds the head of the femur).**

1. An angiography would not be anticipated since it is a diagnostic tool used to study the vascular system. X rays are taken of suspected areas following the administration of a radiopaque contrast agent.

2. Magnetic resonance imaging (MRI) would not be anticipated since it is not as likely to identify more difficult areas of suspected injuries such as the acetabulum. Also, clients with pacemakers, metal implants, and braces are unable to use MRI because of its use of magnetic fields.

4. Arthroscopy would not be anticipated since it requires an invasive operative procedure. It allows for direct visualization of a joint.

Nursing Process: Planning

Client Need: Physiological Integrity

6 - 1 0

③ **You will document your observation as kyphosis (an increased roundness or convexity of the thoracic spinal curve). Kyphosis is often noted in the elderly who are experiencing osteoporosis (loss of bone mass).**

1. Scoliosis (a lateral curving of the thoracic spine) may be congenital, idiopathic (no known cause), or the consequence of injury or disease.

2. Osteoporosis (loss of bone mass) is associated with the aging process. Osteoporosis may contribute to kyphosis.

4. Lordosis (exaggeration of the concave portion of the thoracic spine, or swayback) is normal for the toddler and is also seen in pregnant women, whose center of gravity has changed during pregnancy. Lordosis is considered abnormal when noted in other populations, such as adolescents.

Nursing Process: Assessing

Client Need: Health Promotion and Maintenance

6 - 1 1

① The client is experiencing the inflammatory stage of the bone healing process. During this stage (stage 1), there is bleeding into the injured tissue and the formation of a hematoma, white blood cells begin debridement of dead cells, and the client experiences pain.

2. The cellular proliferation stage occurs within the first 5 days. Fibrin strands begin to form and the interrupted blood supply is recreated. Cartilage and fibrous connective tissue develop.

3. The callus formation stage occurs within the continued growth of the cartilage from each bone fragment. The gap created by the fracture begins to close. After approximately 3 to 4 weeks, the fractured bone fragments will be united.

4. The ossification stage is identified by the formation of bone substance (ossification) and the continued unification of the fracture. This process may take as long as 3 to 4 months. The final remodeling (stage V) of the affected bone may take additional months to years depending on the injury, the bone, and the general healing process.

Nursing Process: Analyzing
Client Need: Physiological Integrity

6 - 1 2

④ You would expect your assessment to reveal numbness of the thumb and first and second fingers. Carpal tunnel syndrome is a neuropathy caused by entrapment of the median nerve at the wrist. Compression occurs due to a thickened flexor tendon sheath, skeletal encroachment, or soft-tissue mass on the median nerve at the wrist. Symptoms include pain, numbness, paresthesia, and possibly weakness along the median nerve (thumb and first and second fingers).

1. A weakened grasp is associated with epicondylitis (tennis elbow).

2. Pain in the shoulder is not associated with carpal tunnel syndrome. Carpal tunnel syndrome affects the wrist.

3. Flexion of the little and ring fingers is seen with Dupuytren's contracture (the ring and little fingers bend into the palm so they cannot be extended).

Nursing Process: Assessing
Client Need: Physiological Integrity

6 - 1 3

① **Asymmetry of the hip with a positive Ortolani's maneuver is indicative of congenital hip dysplasia. Ortolani's maneuver refers to an audible click when reducing a dislocated hip.**

2. Asymmetry of the gluteal folds may be a normal finding but not with a positive Ortolani's maneuver. An Ortolani's maneuver indicates an inability of the hip to fully abduct. The hip is unstable and the femur head actually slides out of the socket.

3. Cerebral palsy may be ruled out by assessing for tight abductor muscles at 4 to 6 weeks old.

4. Deficiency of vitamin D leads to poor bone formation, or rickets, not congenital hip dysplasia.

Nursing Process: Evaluating
Client Need: Physiological Integrity

6 - 1 4

② **You will perform range-of-motion exercises. Exercise is the only preventive measure for contractions. Exercise keeps tendons, ligaments, and muscles flexible. For clients with existing contracture, the exercising is done to the limit of their contractures.**

1. Range of motion may be easier to accomplish after relaxation of the joint in a warm bath, but daily bathing is contraindicated because of the fragile skin of geriatric clients.

3. Turning clients from side to side will not exercise the client's joints.

4. Supporting contracted joints on pillows will provide comfort but worsen the contractures.

Nursing Process: Implementing
Client Need: Physiological Integrity

6 - 1 5

④ **Placing sharp objects under the cast is contraindicated. This can cause skin irritation or breakdown and create a site for infection.**

1. Clients should avoid the use of powder around the cast because it can predispose the skin to irritation, breakdown, and infection.

2. Plastic bags should be used during bathing to protect the cast from moisture.

3. The physician should be notified of any sign of infection under the cast.

Nursing Process: Implementing
Client Need: Health Promotion and Maintenance

6 - 1 6

③ **The physician must be notified immediately. Cold, pale fingers are classic symptoms of compartment syndrome, which is a progressive degeneration of muscles and nerves resulting from severe interruption of blood flow.**

1. Elevation of the extremity is not the primary intervention.
2. Pain relief is important but not the first priority.
4. Range-of-motion exercises are contraindicated for this condition since it will cause the venom to enter the bloodstream more rapidly.

Nursing Process: Evaluating

Client Need: Physiological Integrity

6 - 1 7

① **Small, frequent feedings will prevent discomfort. The nurse should instruct the client about smaller but frequent portions to ensure understanding and cooperation. The nurse will also recommend that the client in a spica cast be placed in a prone position while eating to prevent aspiration.**

2. A 12-year-old would resent smaller portions of food if given only 3 meals a day. Also, the client needs the proper nourishment.
3. Fluids should not be restricted because constipation is a potential problem for clients in a spica cast.
4. Alternating liquids with solids is not realistic. Persons in a spica cast should be served small, bite-size pieces of food. Fluids should be taken through a straw.

Nursing Process: Evaluating

Client Need: Physiological Integrity

6 - 1 8

② **Clients who have bilateral total knee replacements are at high risk for fat embolus during the first 24 to 72 hours postoperatively. Symptoms of fat emboli include confusion, dyspnea, anxiety, and petechiae.**

1. Bowel impaction is common with decreased activity but assessment for bowel impaction would not take priority at this time.
3. Infection is not usually present during the first 3 postoperative days.
4. Assessment for pedal pulses is important but does not take priority over the assessment for fat emboli. A fat embolus is life threatening.

Nursing Process: Assessing

Client Need: Health Promotion and Maintenance

6 - 1 9

② To walk up stairs with crutches, clients with a broken leg would utilize a modified 3-point gait. Clients would start at the bottom of the stairs, transferring their body weight to the crutches. The unaffected leg will be advanced between the crutches to the first stair, the weight will be shifted from the crutches to the unaffected leg, and then the client will align both crutches on the stair. Three points are on the stair at all times.

1. With a 2-point gait, each crutch is moved at the same time as the opposing leg. This requires partial weight bearing on each foot, which would not be possible for a client with a broken leg.

3. A 4-point gait requires weight bearing on both legs. With this gait, each leg is moved alternately with each crutch.

4. The swing-through gait is utilized primarily by paraplegics. The paralyzed legs are supported by braces. With the client's weight supported on the braced legs, the client places the crutches one stride in front and then swings through the crutches while they support the body's weight.

Nursing Process: Implementing
Client Need: Safe, Effective Care Environment

6 - 2 0

③ The walker and the weaker left leg are moved first. The body weight should be borne by the stronger right leg. The stronger leg is moved into the walker while weight is borne by the arms on the walker and the weak leg.

1, 2, and 4. The walker and the weak left leg should be moved first. Body weight should be borne by the stronger leg. The weaker left leg should not be dragged due to the probability of further injury.

Nursing Process: Evaluating
Client Need: Safe, Effective Care Environment

6 - 2 1

① A joint should never be forced beyond its capacity. The nurse should not move the joint past the area where the client might experience discomfort.

2. Exercise should be stopped before the pain occurs. "No pain, no gain" does not apply to range-of-motion exercises.

3. The nurse should support the joint being exercised by holding areas both proximal and distal to the joint.

4. Each movement should be repeated only 5 times.

Nursing Process: Implementing
Client Need: Health Promotion and Maintenance

6-22

① Rehabilitation is necessary after a modified radical mastectomy because underlying tissues are removed. The aim of rehabilitation is to restore use of the affected arm as soon as possible to prevent contractures and muscle shortening, maintain muscle tone, and improve circulation in the arm.

2. Exercising the arm after a modified radical mastectomy will not decrease postoperative pain. Pain will decrease as the incision site heals.

3. Exercise will not eliminate postoperative swelling that occurs at the incision site. Swelling will diminish after the injured cells have healed and normal blood flow returns.

4. Preoperative exercises are performed to teach clients what is expected of them postoperatively when they will be experiencing pain.

Nursing Process: Implementing
Client Need: Health Promotion and Maintenance

6-23

④ Asymmetry in the flank area is indicative of scoliosis. Scoliosis is lateral curvature of the spine.

1, 2, and 3. Scoliosis can be ruled out if the client's head is in alignment with the gluteal fold, there is symmetry of the thoracic area, and both legs are equal in length.

Nursing Process: Analyzing
Client Need: Physiological Integrity

6-24

① The nurse will apply firm pressure to the site of the aspiration for at least 5 minutes. Bone marrow aspiration on adult clients is obtained from the sternum or iliac crest. Because there is a slight risk of hemorrhage, firm pressure is applied over the site of aspiration for approximately 5 minutes. If a bone marrow biopsy is performed from the iliac crest (the sternum is too thin for a biopsy), pressure should be applied for approximately 60 minutes. This is accomplished by having the client lie in a recumbent position on the affected side with a pressure dressing in place.

2, 3, and 4. Applying an adhesive bandage, topical ointments, and ice packs are not procedures that need to be implemented immediately.

Nursing Process: Implementing
Client Need: Physiological Integrity

6 - 2 5

④ **Keeping toys within reach of the child will facilitate maintenance of proper body alignment. Also, the buttocks should be kept slightly off the bed to provide countertraction. The sheets need to be kept clean, dry, and wrinkle-free to prevent skin breakdown.**

1. Turning the child from side to side should be discouraged since the body should be kept in good alignment.
2. The upper body needs to be kept flat to provide sufficient countertraction.
3. Bryant's traction does not utilize pins. It is a type of skin traction.

Nursing Process: Planning
Client Need: Health Promotion and Maintenance

6 - 2 6

① **Traction weight may not be removed without a physician's prescription.**

2. Body alignment should always be maintained.
3. Pain medication should be administered for the client's comfort approximately 30 minutes prior to the procedure.
4. All procedures should be explained to the client.

Nursing Process: Implementing
Client Need: Safe, Effective Care Environment

6 - 2 7

③ **The nurse should walk closely behind and slightly to the side of the client. The greatest degree of safety is provided when the nurse walks behind and slightly to the side of the client. Vulnerability for the client with a walker is at the back where the walker is open. The nurse must be able to see ahead of the client.**

1. Walking directly behind the client will not give the nurse the visibility needed to help the client move forward.
2. Walking in front of the client is contraindicated because the greatest degree of vulnerability for the client is behind the open walker.
4. Walking beside the client does not give the client the support that is needed with the walker being open in the back.

Nursing Process: Implementing
Client Need: Safe, Effective Care Environment

6-28

   ① **Immediately following intermaxillary fixation, the client should be placed in a side-lying position with the head slightly elevated. The side-lying position is the safest following surgery due to the potential for vomiting. Also, slight elevation of the head will facilitate breathing. The ultimate goal is to prevent the aspiration of vomitus. Vomiting may occur following surgery due to inadequate ventilation during anesthesia or to relieve the stomach of mucus and saliva swallowed during anesthesia.**

   2. An upright position (90-degree angle) would be unsafe should the client vomit. Flexing the neck (tilting the chin toward the chest) would interfere with breathing and potentiate aspiration should vomiting occur.

   3. A horizontal recumbent position (lying on the back) is dangerous. Aspiration is likely if the client vomits.

   4. A prone position (lying on the stomach) would interfere with breathing and potentiate aspiration should vomiting occur.

Nursing Process: Implementing
Client Need: Safe, Effective Care Environment

6-29

   ① **Clients should know how to operate the on/off switch of a continuous passive motion machine in case of emergencies.**

   2 and 3. The physician prescribes the flexion and extension movements as well as the speed of the machine. The client should not make any adjustments.

   4. External and internal rotation movements are not available options.

Nursing Process: Planning
Client Need: Safe, Effective Care Environment

6-30

   ① **Rest is very important for the child with juvenile rheumatoid arthritis and would be facilitated by clustering of care. Clustering of care will provide uninterrupted periods of rest.**

   2. Anti-inflammatory medication is more effective than narcotics for control of pain.

   3. High protein and high vitamins are not recommended. The diet needs to be well-balanced.

   4. Heat is more soothing than cool packs to the inflamed joints.

Nursing Process: Planning
Client Need: Health Promotion and Maintenance

6 - 3 1

② **The most likely cause for the client's complaint of numbness is nerve damage or nerve entrapment due to edema, bleeding, or bony fragments.**

1. Blood loss and other injuries may cause hypovolemic shock.

3. Paralysis may be caused by nerve damage. However, the client would be more likely to complain of lack of sensation as opposed to numbness. Untreated nerve damage could cause paralysis.

4. Involuntary muscle contractions (muscle spasms) may occur near the fracture. Pain is experienced as a result of muscle spasms, not numbness.

Nursing Process: Assessing

Client Need: Physiological Integrity

6 - 3 2

④ **To prevent hip dislocation after a total hip replacement, the hip should be kept in abduction and in a neutral rotation to prevent dislocation. This can be accomplished with the use of abductor splints or pillows between the client's legs.**

1, 2, and 3. Crossing the client's legs, placing pillows along the back of the client, and using a drawsheet to facilitate turning could cause a dislocation of the affected hip.

Nursing Process: Implementing

Client Need: Physiological Integrity

6 - 3 3

① **Methylprednisolone (Meprolone) is a glucocorticoid medication. These medications are thought to contribute to the development of osteoporosis because they tend to impair calcium transport, which affects bone density.**

2. Calcium carbonate (Amitone) is used in the treatment or prevention of osteoporosis.

3. Ranitidine (Zantac) is an antiulcer drug and does not affect osteoporosis.

4. Ramipril (Altace) is an angiotensin-converting enzyme (ACE) inhibitor and does not affect bone density.

Nursing Process: Evaluating

Client Need: Health Promotion and Maintenance

6 - 3 4

(1) **An immediate nursing intervention would be to relieve pain. A gouty attack is sudden. The joint is intensely painful, swollen, and extremely tender. Relief of pain is the immediate goal. Narcotics may be used until definitive treatment is established. Colchicine is the drug of choice, but it may take 2 to 24 hours to relieve pain.**

2. Anti-inflammatory agents are administered. These would be given after relief of pain is accomplished.

3. Relieving pressure on the affected joints would be considered after relief of pain.

4. Application of cold packs may be done to reduce inflammation after the relief of pain.

Nursing Process: Implementing
Client Need: Physiological Integrity

6 - 3 5

(2) **The nurse will suspect a fat embolism. A fat embolism is caused by a globule of fat entering a torn or lacerated blood vessel and causing an obstruction. A fat embolism is a complication that may occur following a fracture of the pelvis or a long bone. Onset is within 72 hours of trauma or other insult.**

1. Symptoms of nerve damage would include persistent localized pain, numbness, tingling, and motor weakness not previously present.

3. Symptoms of hypostatic pneumonia would include chest pain, fever, productive cough, dyspnea, headache, and fatigue.

4. Dyspnea, restlessness, tachycardia, progressive cyanosis, and mental confusion are not related to paralysis.

Nursing Process: Analyzing
Client Need: Physiological Integrity

6 - 3 6

(1) **The wheelchair should be placed on the left side of the bed where the equipment is located. The wheelchair needs to be facing the head of the bed so the client can reach for the chair arm with the uninvolved strong arm and help with the transfer.**

2 and 4. The wheelchair needs to be on the left side of the bed. If the wheelchair could be placed on the right side of the bed, then it would need to be placed facing the foot of the bed to facilitate transfer from the bed to the chair.

3. With the wheelchair facing the foot of the bed, the client would not be able to reach with the uninvolved arm to grasp the wheelchair.

Nursing Process: Implementing
Client Need: Safe, Effective Care Environment

6 - 3 7

② **The client's request for assistance in placing a waterproof petal around the edges of the cast demonstrates interest in keeping the cast in good condition.**

1. Whittling at the cast is a way of defacing it. Damaging a cast indicates the child has not accepted it.

3. Stuffing paper in the cast is viewed by the child as a possible reason to remove it.

4. Refusing to go to the playroom may indicate that the client is embarrassed to be seen by others.

Nursing Process: Evaluating
Client Need: Psychosocial Integrity

6 - 3 8

③ **The swing-through gait is used by clients who have paralysis of the legs and hips. Both crutches are moved forward together. The client then lifts the body weight with the arms and swings through and beyond the crutches.**

1. To use the 4-point gait, the client would need to bear weight on both legs.

2. The 3-point gait would require weight bearing on one unaffected leg.

4. The 2-point gait requires partial weight bearing on both legs.

Nursing Process: Planning
Client Need: Physiological Integrity

6 - 3 9

④ **Traction is not applied to provide for comfort. In fact, traction is often uncomfortable.**

1, 2, and 3. When a client is placed in 90-90 traction for a fractured femur, the purpose of the traction is to reduce dislocation, immobilize the leg, and decrease muscle spasms. Traction can realign the bone, prevent deformity, maintain alignment, and provide rest for the extremity.

Nursing Process: Implementing
Client Need: Physiological Integrity

6 - 4 0

② **The vastus lateralis is the preferred site for an intramuscular injection in infants. This muscle is best developed and relatively free of blood vessels and major nerves.**

1. The deltoid muscle is not large enough in an infant for intramuscular injection and would probably cause an abcess.

3. The dorsogluteal muscle is not as large as the vastus lateralis in an infant. The dorsogluteal can be used for intramuscular injections when the child has been walking for approximately 1 year and the muscle has developed.

4. The ventrogluteal muscle will not be developed enough for intramuscular injections until a child is approximately 18 months of age.

Nursing Process: Analyzing

Client Need: Health Promotion and Maintenance

6 - 4 1

③ **Fever and complaints of fatigue are common manifestations seen in clients who are experiencing acute rheumatoid arthritis. With an acute onset of rheumatoid arthritis, numerous joints suddenly become painful and swollen and the client also experiences chills and prostration.**

1, 2, and 4. Pedal edema, generalized erythema, bradycardia, and slow respirations are not common manifestations of rheumatoid arthritis.

Nursing Process: Assessing

Client Need: Physiological Integrity

6 - 4 2

② **Inadequate blood supply may occur following a dislocation and lack of blood supply will cause necrosis if the dislocation is not treated.**

1. Shock is not likely to occur following a dislocation. However, hypovolemic shock is a potential problem when bone fragments and lacerated vessels are involved.

3. Fat embolism is a complication of fractured bones, not dislocations.

4. It is not until after dislocation has been reduced that attention is turned toward tissue healing and the prevention of contractures.

Nursing Process: Evaluation

Client Need: Health Promotion and Maintenance

6 - 4 3

① A client who has had an above-the-knee (AK) amputation should have the affected limb placed in a position of extension to prevent contracture.

2, 3, and 4. Flexion, internal rotation, and external rotation will lead to the development of contractures in the affected limb.

Nursing Process: Implementing
Client Need: Health Promotion and Maintenance

6 - 4 4

① The nurse will anticipate a prescription for the tensilon test. Myasthenia gravis is caused by an inadequate amount of acetylcholine at the myoneural junction. Administration of edrophonium (Tensilon), a short-acting cholinesterase inhibitor, can help to diagnose myasthenia gravis. When the client's strength improves after receiving Tensilon, the diagnosis of myasthenia gravis is confirmed.

2. A cold stimulation test may be scheduled to confirm Raynaud's syndrome, not myasthenia gravis.

3. Magnetic resonance imaging is helpful in confirming the diagnoses of cerebral infarction, tumor, abscess, edema, hemorrhage, nerve fiber damage, and demyelination, not myasthenia gravis.

4. Electroencephalography is valuable in assessing clients with symptoms of brain tumors, abscesses, and cerebral damage.

Nursing Process: Assessing
Client Need: Physiological Integrity

Practice Test 7

Neurological System and Special Senses/Pain

7 - 1

Which of these observations would be considered characteristic of a normal newborn?

1. random, jerky, uneven movements of the eyes
2. a high-pitched, shrill cry
3. bulging fontanels
4. a lethargic posture during a bath

7 - 2

After a lumbar disectomy, postoperative discharge instructions are prescribed. Which one of the following situations would the client be instructed to report to the surgeon immediately?

1. drainage from the operative site
2. discomfort for the first 2 weeks postoperatively
3. continuing to be overweight
4. diminished sexual activity

7 - 3

Which of the following medications is useful in the treatment of Parkinson's disease?

1. vasopressin
2. levodopa
3. aminophylline
4. levothyroxine

7 - 4

A client with cancer is complaining of pain in the back. Which question will assess the severity of the client's pain?

1. "Do you have more pain in your back than you do in any other area of your body?"
2. "Did your pain begin in your back or did it originate elsewhere?"
3. "Would you say your pain is worse when you are in a sitting position or when you are lying down?"
4. "On a scale of 0 to 10 with 0 being no pain and 10 being a lot of pain, what is your pain?"

7 - 5

A client is admitted to the hospital with a ruptured lumbar intervertebral disc. Prescriptions include bed rest, moist, warm heat packs, and meperidine hydrochloride. Before applying moist heat to the client's lower back, it is essential for the nurse to take which of the following actions?

1. Place a plastic protective covering on the skin before applying the heat source.
2. Apply a thin layer of petrolatum jelly on the skin before applying the heat source.
3. Check the temperature of the heat source.
4. Wrap the heat source in a towel.

7 - 6

A 3-month-old infant with hydrocephalus had a ventriculoperitoneal shunt replacement yesterday. The infant is irritable and you note the dressing on the infant's head is wet. Possible sources might be perspiration, saliva, emesis, or cerebrospinal fluid. To distinguish if the drainage is from cerebrospinal fluid, you will test the fluid for:

1. pH.
2. chloride.
3. bacteria via culture.
4. glucose.

7 - 7

A newborn is diagnosed with hydrocephalus. Which of the following measures should the nurse include in the care plan?

1. Measure the abdominal girth daily.
2. Change the infant's position every 2 hours.
3. Feed the infant on an established schedule.
4. Place the infant so the head is lower than the rest of the body.

7 - 8

Your client has Alzheimer's disease and frequently becomes agitated. Which of the following measures would be best to include in the client's plan of care?

1. Keep the client's room dimly lit, the side rails up, and stimulation at a minimum.
2. Place the client in a wheelchair at the nurses' station and give small simple tasks that are repetitious in nature.
3. Apply restraints and monitor the client daily.
4. Move the client close to the nurses' station, turn on a radio to soothing music, and check the client frequently.

7 - 9

A professional football player is hospitalized following a cervical 6 injury to the spinal cord. The client was placed on a mechanical ventilator immediately after the injury and is in skeletal traction. During the first 24 hours after the injury, the priority nursing diagnosis is:

1. impaired skin integrity.
2. decreased cardiac output.
3. ineffective individual coping.
4. impaired gas exchange.

7 - 1 0

A client has a grand mal seizure. A prescription for 1000 mg phenytoin intravenously is to be given. You will:

1. give the medication in a rapid intravenous push.
2. give concurrent nitroglycerin for the anticipated hypertension.
3. mix the medications in D5NS.
4. monitor the pulse and blood pressure throughout the infusion.

7 - 1 1

A 69-year-old client has Parkinson's disease and is admitted to a long-term care facility. Admission prescriptions include diet and activity as tolerated. Prior to developing the client's nursing-care plan, to which of these measures should the nurse give priority?

1. Explain to the client the roles of various nursing personnel.
2. Introduce the client to other long-term ambulatory clients.
3. Find out about the client's routines for care at home.
4. Evaluate how much the client knows about Parkinson's disease.

7 - 1 2

Which of the following observations by the nurse would indicate increased intracranial pressure in a client?

1. oliguria
2. pallor
3. lethargy
4. hypothermia

7 - 1 3

A client who is experiencing intractable pain in the head, neck, and arms may have which of the following procedures performed in order to relieve the pain?

1. cingulotomy
2. cordotomy
3. thalamotomy
4. rhizotomy

7 - 1 4

When talking to the parents of a child recently diagnosed with epilepsy, the most appropriate statement is:

1. "Medications used to treat seizures may cause problems with behavior."
2. "Your child should be able to participate in extracurricular activities."
3. "Be careful, since children die from head injuries during seizures."
4. "Avoid making your child cry since that can cause a seizure."

7 - 1 5

A client is diagnosed with herpes zoster involving the trigeminal nerve on the right side of the face. The client complains of itchiness on the right side of the face. Which procedure should the nurse include in the plan of care?

1. applying cool compresses
2. cleansing the area tid
3. removing any scales that may appear
4. applying petrolatum jelly qid

7 - 1 6

A child has tympanostomy ventilating tubes surgically implanted in both ears. Which of the following is an especially important preventive measure against infection following the insertion of the tubes?

1. Clean ear canals with alcohol solution daily.
2. Use earplugs when swimming or bathing.
3. Blow bubbles daily to keep the tubes patent.
4. Administer a mild decongestant.

7 - 1 7

A client has been hospitalized for an acute exacerbation of multiple sclerosis and is to be discharged on prednisone. The client has been instructed to continue taking the medication for 4 more weeks. The nurse is planning discharge teaching about the medication. Which instruction is essential for the client to know about prednisone?

1. The dosage of prednisone should be tapered off gradually.
2. The client is to take the same dose each day until the prescription is finished.
3. The drug should be taken before meals on an empty stomach.
4. The client will need to increase salt intake to prevent sodium depletion.

7 - 1 8

Assessment of a 30-year-old client reveals a positive Babinski reflex. What does this assessment indicate?

1. cerebellar dysfunction
2. increased intracranial pressure
3. central nervous system disease of the motor system
4. interruption of the peripheral nervous system

7-19

Which medication would be the drug of choice for a client experiencing a grand mal seizure?

1. ativan
2. dilantin
3. clonopin
4. prednisone

7-20

During your morning assessment of a client with paraplegia, you notice a marked increase in blood pressure. Your client complains of a headache and blurred vision. You notice that your client's upper body and head are diaphoretic. An appropriate intervention would be to:

1. administer acetaminophen po for the headache and explain that this is inevitable in a paraplegic.
2. reassure the client that this is a typical emotional response to stress.
3. quickly and vigorously palpate the chest and abdomen for any nodules.
4. assist the client to a sitting position very slowly and notify the physician.

7-21

A 9-year-old is admitted to the pediatric unit. Both eyes are bandaged because of an accidental eye injury. The child is scheduled for surgery the next day. The client's plan of care is least likely to include instructions:

1. for all personnel to speak as they enter the child's room.
2. allowing the child to take a favorite stuffed toy to the operating room.
3. to explain about equipment in use such as the intravenous infusion.
4. to explain what the operating room will look like.

7-22

Which of the following medications would be administered for the treatment of tonic-clonic seizure activity?

1. valproate
2. ranitidine
3. digoxin
4. captopril

7 - 2 3

A newly admitted client has a hearing impairment. Which nursing intervention will be the most useful in helping the nurse to communicate?

1. Use visual cues.
2. Refer the client to the speech therapist.
3. Speak slowly and articulate clearly.
4. Allow time for understanding and a response.

7 - 2 4

A client with hyperthyroidism is experiencing exophthalmos. Which nursing intervention is appropriate?

1. Keep the head of the bed flat.
2. Provide a high-calorie diet.
3. Instill methylcellulose eyedrops qid.
4. Place the client in a room close to the nurses' station.

7 - 2 5

Your client is experiencing severe depression that has not been alleviated by medication. The client is scheduled for electroconvulsive therapy. Nursing interventions appropriate for this therapy include:

1. informing the client that post-procedure memory loss is permanent.
2. discussing with the client and family that only 1 treatment may be given safely in a month.
3. describing the intended cardiac arrhythmias, including ventricular fibrillation, which occur during these treatments.
4. monitoring vital signs and airway patency after the treatment.

7 - 2 6

Your client has a head injury and is exhibiting signs of diabetes insipidus. Because of this development, you know you must monitor this client very closely for:

1. agitation and confabulation.
2. congestive heart failure.
3. hyperglycemia and metabolic acidosis.
4. dehydration and hypovolemia.

7 - 2 7

The following preoperative medications are prescribed for a child: meperidine 8 mg; atropine sulfate 0.06 mg. The medications are available as follows: meperidine 50 mg/cc; atropine sulfate 0.40 mg/cc. To administer the prescribed doses, the nurse should prepare:

1. meperidine 0.16 cc and atropine 0.15 cc.
2. meperidine 0.26 cc and atropine 0.20 cc.
3. meperidine 1 minim and atropine 3 minims.
4. meperidine 2 minims and atropine 4 minims.

7 - 2 8

To assess for blockage in the vertebral canal, the Queckenstedt test was performed during a lumbar puncture procedure. A rapid rise in cerebrospinal fluid pressure while pressing the neck veins indicates:

1. a blockage is present in the vertebral canal.
2. the presence of a tumor in the vertebral canal.
3. infections such as meningitis.
4. a normal finding.

7 - 2 9

A client with a spinal cord injury has a nursing diagnosis of "impaired physical mobility related to central nervous system injury." Your goal is to have the client gain mobility within the limits imposed by the injury. What assessment finding indicates that this goal has been met?

1. skin dry and intact
2. absence of contractures
3. seeks diversional activity
4. relaxed facial expression

7 - 3 0

You are using the Glasgow Coma Scale as part of your assessment for a client with a head injury. During your assessment, you observe the following: Eyes open to speech, motor response appropriate, client obeys commands, conversation is confused. You will assign the client a score of:

1. 1 to 2.
2. 4 to 5.
3. 12 to 13.
4. 19 to 20.

7 - 3 1

A client diagnosed with acute hypothyroidism has just sustained a fracture
of the left humerus. Morphine sulfate is
prescribed for pain. The prescription reads:
morphine sulfate 5 mg intramuscularly every
6 hours prn for pain. In response to your
client's complaint of pain, the most appropriate action would be to:

1. administer the morphine as prescribed.
2. notify the physician and discuss non-
   narcotic options.
3. administer no analgesia.
4. administer the morphine intravenously
   because it will act faster.

7 - 3 2

A 76-year-old has cataracts in both eyes and
is scheduled through the day surgery clinic
for a left cataract extraction. Instillation of
mydriatic drops is prescribed preoperatively.
Preoperative assessment of the client's vision
by the nurse would reveal which of the
following findings?

1. loss of visual acuity
2. the presence of double vision
3. complaints of visual fatigue
4. presence of floating filaments

7 - 3 3

A client was admitted to your unit with a
medical diagnosis of cerebrovascular accident. You are concerned about your client
developing increased intracranial pressure.
What assessment finding is an early indication of this occurrence?

1. drowsiness
2. vomiting
3. hemiplegia
4. widened pulse pressure

7 - 3 4

An adult client complains of having periodic
episodes of blindness in the right eye. The
physician is concerned that the oculomotor
nerve has been damaged. Which assessment
technique will verify this?

1. Inspect the retina with an ophthalmoscope.
2. Assess visual acuity with the Snellen chart.
3. Shine a penlight directly into the right eye
   and then observe pupillary response.
4. Shine a penlight on the bridge of the nose
   and note where the reflection is on each
   eye.

7 - 3 5

Which of these findings would not be suggestive of otitis media in your 3-year-old client?

1. tugging at the earlobe
2. temperature of 104°F
3. pain behind the ear
4. turning the head from side to side

7 - 3 6

A 5-year-old child is admitted with a possible cerebellar brain tumor. Response to which of the following neurological tests is most likely to be abnormal preoperatively?

1. pupil reflexes
2. deep tendon reflexes
3. number recall test
4. standing balance

7 - 3 7

A 6-year-old child with hydrocephalus is admitted for possible ventriculoperitoneal shunt revision. The most likely assessment finding would be:

1. sunset eyes.
2. diplopia.
3. Macewen sign.
4. high-pitched cry.

7 - 3 8

An infant born with a myelomeningocele experienced a successful closure soon after birth. The child is now 15 months old. The most appropriate nursing diagnosis at this time is:

1. altered urinary elimination.
2. impaired verbal communications.
3. bowel incontinence.
4. altered growth and development, gross motor.

7-39

A client had a laminectomy performed under general anesthesia. After recovery, the client is returned to the unit. Vital signs include blood pressure 130/80, pulse rate 80 beats per minute. Which of the following vital signs would indicate the development of shock?

1. blood pressure 100/60, pulse 120
2. blood pressure 120/80, pulse 74
3. blood pressure 140/100, pulse 100
4. blood pressure 150/90, pulse 60

7-40

An infant is diagnosed with bacterial meningitis. Which of the following nursing interventions would be most appropriate at this time?

1. measure weight and head circumference on each shift
2. monitor behavior at each encounter
3. evaluate Kernig's sign each shift
4. monitor fontanel tenseness daily

7-41

A client who has experienced a battery acid splash on the face and in the eyes should first have the eyes treated immediately with:

1. copious water irrigation.
2. sodium bicarbonate irrigation.
3. lidocaine ointment.
4. atropine sulfate solution.

7-42

The most appropriate assessment to perform on a preschool-age child admitted for a possible brain tumor is:

1. walking ability.
2. head circumference.
3. skin color and capillary refill.
4. vocabulary size and use.

7 - 4 3

A client comes to the Emergency Department with slurred speech and a sudden onset of left-sided weakness. Prior to the administration of heparin sodium intravenous, a computer tomography of the head is prescribed. A lumbar puncture is also to be performed after the results of the computer tomography came back as "inconclusive for cerebral bleed." You know that the purpose of the lumbar puncture is to:

1. relieve pressure on the brain by draining cerebral spinal fluid.
2. test for fungal infection.
3. allow for the administration of the heparin sodium.
4. test for the presence of blood.

7 - 4 4

A 75-year-old is seen at a local clinic and receives a diagnosis of herpes zoster involving the trigeminal nerve on the right side of the face. The client has vesicles and a rash on the right cheek. Prescriptions include acetaminophen. In developing a nursing assessment of the client, it would be important for the nurse to obtain the answer to which of the following questions?

1. Has the client been exposed to anyone with chicken pox?
2. Does the client have a history of developing canker sores?
3. Is the client using a new shaving cream?
4. Has the client ever had a dermatologic reaction to food?

7 - 4 5

Which of the following approaches would be most appropriate for the nurse to include in a care plan for a client who is experiencing organic brain syndrome?

1. Carry out activities in the same order each day.
2. Encourage the client to focus conversation on present events.
3. Provide a variety of activities for the client.
4. Introduce the client to all the nursing staff.

7 - 4 6

A client has right-sided homonymous hemianopsia. How will you help the client cope with this deficit?

1. Approach the client from the right side at all times.
2. Place all objects on the right side of the client's bed.
3. Teach the client to turn the head toward the right.
4. Teach the client how to use the left hand to move the right arm.

7 - 4 7

A client with a seizure disorder is scheduled for an electroencephalogram in the morning. What nursing action, if any, is appropriate prior to the examination?

1. Withhold diazepam for 4 hours.
2. Nothing by mouth for 12 hours.
3. Omit coffee for 24 hours.
4. No special nursing actions are needed.

7 - 4 8

Which nursing action can help keep intra-cranial pressure down?

1. Keep the head of the bed flat.
2. Place a pillow under the knees.
3. Encourage deep breaths.
4. Administer 5% dextrose in water at 50 cc per hour.

7 - 4 9

Your pediatric client has otitis media. Amoxicillin is prescribed 20 mg/kg po daily in 3 divided doses every 8 hours. Your client weighs 60 lbs. How much of the medication will 1 dose contain?

1. 18 g
2. 180 mg
3. 36 g
4. 360 mg

7 - 5 0

Which prescription would you question for a client who has a diagnosis of acute hemorrhagic stroke?

1. dipyridamole 25 mg po daily
2. diazepam 10 mg prn intravenously for agitation
3. phenytoin sodium 100 mg po tid
4. dexamethasone 60 mg intravenously every 6 hours

7 - 5 1

Upon arrival at the Emergency Department, a client experiences diminished touch sensation in the lower extremities following a motor vehicle accident. The nurse should anticipate and assess related neurological deficits that include:

1. pupil size and reaction.
2. distension of the urinary bladder.
3. respiratory distress.
4. presence of headache and nausea.

7 - 5 2

A newborn with a myelomeningocele is to have a surgical repair 24 to 48 hours post birth. The most important ongoing assessment in the preoperative period is for:

1. fontanel status.
2. hip dysplasia.
3. bowel incontinence.
4. pain sensation below the defect.

Practice Test 7

Answers, Rationales, and Explanations

7 - 1

① **Random, jerky, uneven movements of the eyes (nystagmus) is a normal finding in the newborn, who has not learned to focus.**

2. A high-pitched, shrill cry is associated with neurological disorder.

3. Bulging fontanels are associated with increased intracranial pressure.

4. A lethargic posture during a bath is associated with a central nervous system disorder. The infant should have symmetric movement and strength in all extremities.

Nursing Process: Assessing
Client Need: Health Promotion and Maintenance

7 - 2

① **The client should be told to report any drainage from the operative site immediately. Drainage may indicate infection and needs immediate attention.**

2. Discomfort for the first 2 weeks should be brought to the attention of the surgeon, but it is not the immediate concern.

3. There is no indication that the client is overweight.

4. Diminished sexual activity can be addressed later.

Nursing Process: Implementing
Client Need: Health Promotion and Maintenance

7 - 3

② **The medication that is most useful in the treatment of Parkinson's disease is levodopa. Parkinson's disease is caused by a degeneration of a portion of the nervous system. Levodopa (L-Dopa) augments the body's dopamine level. Dopamine is essential for neurotransmission.**

1. Vasopressin (ADH) is an antidiuretic hormone replacement and has no impact on neurotransmission.

3. Aminophylline (Somophyllin) is a bronchodilator and has no impact on neurotransmission.

4. Levothyroxine (Levothroid) is a hormone replacement and has no impact on neurotransmission.

Nursing Process: Evaluating
Client Need: Physiological Integrity

7 - 4

④ **Asking the client to evaluate pain on a 0 to 10 scale will help to identify the severity of the pain.**

1. Asking the client if there is more pain in the back than any other place in the body will identify the location of the pain, not the severity of the pain.

2. Asking if the pain began in the back or some other area will identify the origin of the pain, not the severity of the pain.

3. Asking the client if the pain is worse when sitting or lying down will help to identify aggravating factors, not the severity of the pain.

Nursing Process: Assessing

Client Need: Safe, Effective Care Environment

7 - 5

③ **The nurse should check the temperature of the heat source (moist pack) before application. If the heat source is too hot, it may burn the client. Warm, moist heat packs are applied (10 to 20 minutes) to the lower back several times a day to relax spastic muscles.**

1. Once a moist compress is applied to the client's lower back, it should be covered with a piece of plastic to retain the heat.

2. Petrolatum jelly is applied to the skin if the compress solution is irritating to tissues. This client's compresses are moist, warm heat packs and would not be irritating to the skin.

4. Warm, moist heat packs are not wrapped in a towel. An example of a heat source that should be wrapped in a towel would be a hot-water bottle.

Nursing Process: Implementing

Client Need: Physiological Integrity

7 - 6

④ **To distinguish if the drainage is cerebrospinal fluid, the nurse will test for glucose. Glucose is present in cerebrospinal fluid (CSF) but not in perspiration and saliva. Because the infant is only 1 day postoperative, there will be no food in the stomach to test positive for glucose in emesis.**

1. The pH of CSF is not very distinct in comparison to many other body fluids except stomach contents. Because the infant is only 1 day postoperative, there will be no food in the stomach to test positive for glucose.

2. Chloride level is not a marker of CSF.

3. A culture could only grow organisms and this would not help to identify what the drainage is.

Nursing Process: Planning

Client Need: Health Promotion and Maintenance

7 - 7

② **The nursing-care plan for a child with hydrocephalus will include changing the infant's position every 2 hours. It is important to change the infant's position at regular intervals to prevent the development of pressure areas on the baby's head.**

1. The infant's head circumference, not abdominal girth, should be measured at least once a day. Measurements should be recorded and plotted on a graph.

3. The infant's feeding schedule should be flexible enough to accommodate diagnostic procedures.

4. Placing the infant's head lower than the body will increase intracranial pressure and is contraindicated.

Nursing Process: Planning
Client Need: Health Promotion and Maintenance

7 - 8

④ **The client should be moved closer to the nurses' station, where frequent checks can be made and soothing music can be heard. Current thoughts on Alzheimer's disease indicate that overstimulation increases agitation in clients. Yet stimulation is necessary to provide some reality orientation.**

1. Clients with Alzheimer's should be placed in brightly lighted rooms during the day and sufficient light at night to help identify surroundings.

2. Placing the client in a wheelchair will limit mobility and can increase agitation. Having the client engage in repetitious tasks is not recommended because of the short attention span.

3. Restraints are not recommended. They tend to increase agitation.

Nursing Process: Planning
Client Need: Psychosocial Integrity

7 - 9

④ **During the first 24 hours after a cervical injury, maintenance of adequate respiratory function is critical to survival. Oxygen is administered to maintain a high arterial PO_2 since anoxemia can create or worsen neurological damage to the spinal cord.**

1. The client probably does not have significantly impaired skin integrity at this time. Measures need to be started to prevent skin breakdown, but this is not the priority.

2. Although decreased cardiac output is important, you must first of all have oxygen for the heart to circulate blood around the body.

3. The client is understandably frightened and attempting to cope with the enormity of the injuries. This must be dealt with, but first you must make sure that the client survives the injury.

Nursing Process: Analyzing
Client Need: Physiological Integrity

7-10

④ **Clients receiving intravenous phenytoin (Dilantin) should be monitored for brady-cardia and hypotension. These are two frequently occurring side effects associated with this medication.**

1. The rate of administration of phenytoin should not exceed 50 mg/min.

2. Phenytoin (Dilantin) intravenously may cause hypotension, not hypertension.

3. This medication is to be mixed with normal saline only. Mixing Dilantin with other solutions will cause precipitation.

Nursing Process: Implementing

Client Need: Physiological Integrity

7-11

③ **Before developing a nursing-care plan for a client hospitalized with Parkinson's disease, the nurse should determine what the client's routines are for care at home. The nurse will want to simulate these as much as possible. This will minimize anxiety generated by unexpected routines or demands. Interviewing the client is one method of collecting data for the development of the nursing-care plan. The client is usually the best source for information about patterns of coping with the activities of daily living.**

1. The nurse should explain the roles of various nursing personnel to all clients, not just those with Parkinson's disease.

2. Introducing the client to other long-term ambulatory clients will not influence the development of a nursing-care plan.

4. How much the client knows about Parkinsonism is not likely to affect the nursing-care plan. However, knowing the client's daily home routine of care will be most helpful since the nurse will simulate these routines.

Nursing Process: Assessing

Client Need: Safe, Effective Care Environment

7-12

③ **Lethargy is a sign of increased intracranial pressure that may be observed by the nurse. Other clinical signs of increased intracranial pressure include headache; vomiting; decrease in level of consciousness, motor function, and respirations; abnormal eye movements; changes in pupil size and reaction to light; widening pulse; bradycardia; irregular respiratory pattern; and decreases in motor functioning.**

1, 2, and 4. Oliguria, pallor, and hypothermia are not associated with increased intracranial pressure.

Nursing Process: Analyzing

Client Need: Physiological Integrity

7 - 1 3

③ **Clients experiencing intractable pain in the head, neck, and arms may have a thalamotomy (a surgical technique designed to selectively destroy specific groups of cells in the thalamus for relief of pain).**

1. A cingulotomy (frontal white matter interruption) is performed on clients with intractable pain associated with an extreme psychogenic component.

2. A cordotomy is performed by interrupting the lateral spinothalamic tract in either the cervical or thoracic areas. It may be used to relieve the severe pain associated with terminal cancer.

4. A rhizotomy is performed for traumatic nerve injury. Surgery is performed to interrupt the posterior roots as they enter the spinal cord proximally to the posterior cell. This interrupts the cranial nerve at its entrance into the brain stem. This surgery is used to control the severe chest pain of lung cancer and for pain relief involving head and neck malignancies.

Nursing Process: Evaluating

Client Need: Physiological Integrity

7 - 1 4

② **An appropriate statement to make to the parents of a child recently diagnosed with epilepsy would include the need for the child to continue participating in all activities.**

1. Medications used to treat seizures may cause drowsiness at first but that will soon subside.

3. Telling parents that children die from head injuries during seizures is inappropriate. The parents should be taught to take precautions but should not be taught in such a way that they fear for their child's life.

4. Disciplinary problems could occur as a consequence of the nurse telling parents that they should avoid making their child cry because crying may cause a seizure. Crying rarely precipitates a seizure.

Nursing Process: Implementing

Client Need: Health Promotion and Maintenance

7 - 1 5

① The application of cool compresses is recommended for clients with herpes zoster who are experiencing itchiness. Herpes zoster (shingles) is an infection caused by the reactivation of the varicella virus in clients who have experienced chicken pox. Acyclovir (Zovirax) is an antiviral medication frequently administered to treat this condition. Treatment focuses on relief of pain and avoidance of complications. The nursing-care plan should include the application of cool compresses to the affected area. Cool compresses will relieve the itching, burning, and stabbing pain of herpes zoster by contracting the blood vessels.

2. Cleansing the affected area is not recommended since touching causes pain.

3. Scales are not associated with herpes zoster.

4. Applying petrolatum jelly to the affected area is not recommended due to the potential for spreading the virus.

Nursing Process: Planning
Client Need: Physiological Integrity

7 - 1 6

② The use of earplugs for a child with tympanostomy ventilating tubes can defend against infection by preventing water from entering the external ear canal and going into the middle ear. Contaminated lake and bath water in the ear canal increases the risk for infection.

1. An effective treatment for preventing otitis externa is to place a combination of white vinegar and rubbing alcohol (50/50) in the ear canals in the morning, at night, and after swimming. However, this treatment is not recommended following tube insertion.

3. Having the child "blow bubbles" will increase pressure in the eustachian tube, which in turn will increase the pressure in the middle ear and possibly disrupt the integrity of the tympanostomy tubes.

4. There is no strong link between the use of mild decongestants and the prevention of infection following the implantation of tympanostomy ventilating tubes.

Nursing Process: Implementing
Client Need: Health Promotion and Maintenance

7 - 1 7

① Discharge instructions for clients receiving prednisone should emphasize the need to taper off the use of prednisone gradually. Abrupt discontinuation of prednisone could lead to adrenal insufficiency. Prednisone is a type of hormone whose production and release is normally mandated by the adrenal gland. When exogenous prednisone is taken, usually for more than 2 weeks, the adrenal gland ceases its own release. Therefore, abrupt cessation leads to extreme steroid imbalance until the adrenal gland can resume its normal course.

2. Rapid withdrawal of the drug could lead to adrenal insufficiency and should be avoided.

3. Prednisone causes gastrointestinal irritation and gastric ulcers. It should be taken with food.

4. Prednisone causes potassium (K) depletion and sodium (Na) retention. A Na-restricted diet with potassium supplements should be prescribed for clients receiving prednisone.

Nursing Process: Implementing
Client Need: Health Promotion and Maintenance

7 - 1 8

③ A positive Babinski reflex in a 30-year-old client indicates a central nervous system disease of the motor system. The Babinski reflex is normally seen in infants under the age of six months. The Babinski reflex is characterized by the extension of the great toe and the spreading out of the outer toes when the lateral aspect of the sole is stroked.

1. Cerebellar dysfunction would be manifested by ataxia and incoordination.

2. Increased intracranial pressure (ICP) is manifested by changes in level of consciousness (LOC), increased blood pressure, and decreased heart rate.

4. Interruption of the peripheral nervous system is manifested by numbness, tingling, and possible loss of sensation.

Nursing Process: Analyzing
Client Need: Physiological Integrity

7 - 1 9

② Phenytoin (Dilantin) is the drug of choice for the treatment of grand mal seizures.

1. Lorazepam (Ativan) is indicated when the client is experiencing status epilepticus.

3. Clonazepam (Clonopin) is utilized for absence (petit mal).

4. Prednisone (Meticorten) is an anti-inflammatory corticosteroid preparation and has no impact on seizures.

Nursing Procedure: Planning
Client Need: Physiological Integrity

7-20

④ Appropriate interventions for a client experiencing autonomic dysreflexia would include assisting the client to a sitting position and notifying the physician. This client is exhibiting the classic signs of autonomic dysreflexia that is caused by the stimulation of the nerves below the level of the spinal injury. This may cause cardiac arrhythmias and can be life threatening. By having the client sit up, the extreme hypertension associated with this condition is decreased momentarily until the physician can be notified and an appropriate medication such as diazole (Hyperstat) can be given.

1. Although acetaminophen may treat headaches, this client is exhibiting classic signs of autonomic dysreflexia that require immediate attention.

2. This client is exhibiting the classic signs of autonomic dysreflexia.

3. This client is exhibiting the classic signs of autonomic dysreflexia. Palpating the chest and abdomen would be inappropriate.

Nursing Process: Implementing

Client Need: Physiological Integrity

7-21

④ The least likely plan of care for a child scheduled for surgery who cannot see would be an explanation that describes the operating room. Because the child is unable to see, explaining what the operating room looks like is unimportant. Explaining the sounds, smells, and kinesthetics would be important.

1. Speaking as you enter the room will let the child know someone is present. This will minimize fear and establish mutual respect and trust.

2. Having a security item such as a stuffed toy is very important during traumatic situations for toddlers, preschoolers, and young school-age children.

3. Equipment that can be sensed by the senses other than vision should be explained.

Nursing Process: Planning

Client Need: Psychosocial Integrity

7-22

① Valproate (Depakote) is a medication that may be administered to treat tonic-clonic seizure activity. Depakote is an anticonvulsant medication whose impact on neural transmission makes it a very effective anticonvulsant agent.

2. Ranitidine (Zantac) is an anti-ulcer medication.

3. Digoxin (Lanoxin) is a cardiac glycoside.

4. Captopril (Capoten) is an antihypertensive.

Nursing Process: Planning

Client Need: Physiological Integrity

7-23

③ For the hearing-impaired client, it is imperative that the nurse speak slowly, articulate clearly, and allow time for understanding and a response. The nurse should also speak toward the client's best ear, reduce background noise, and make sure, if the client is wearing a hearing aid, that it is functioning properly.

1. Visual cues are not necessary if the nurse speaks slowly and distinctly.
2. There is no reason to refer the client to a speech therapist. The problem has to do with the client hearing the nurse.
4. The nurse should always allow clients, including the hearing-impaired, time to consider what has been said before expecting a response.

Nursing Process: Implementing
Client Need: Health Promotion and Maintenance

7-24

③ Administration of methylcellulose eye drops qid helps reduce eye irritation for clients who have exophthalmos. Protrusion of the eyeballs (exophthalmos) occurs with hyperthyroidism due to increased deposits of fats and fluid in the retro-orbital tissues. Because of this, there is a potential for injury to the cornea due to dryness and irritation.

1. To prevent increased intraocular pressure, the head of the bed should be elevated, not flat.
2. A high-calorie diet would be appropriate in meeting the client's increasing needs for calories, but would not affect exophthalmos.
4. Clients with hyperthyroidism do not need the additional stimuli that would be experienced by placing them in a high-traffic area.

Nursing Process: Implementing
Client Need: Health Promotion and Maintenance

7-25

④ The nurse will monitor the client's airway patency and vital signs following an electroconvulsive treatment. Nursing interventions prior to electroconvulsive therapy include the administration of a sedative. Therefore, monitoring vital signs and airway patency after the treatment is essential.

1. Memory loss is common, though transient.
2. Treatments may be given 3 times a week.
3. No cardiac arrhythmia is intended.

Nursing Process: Implementing
Client Need: Safe, Effective Care Environment

7 - 2 6

④ **The nurse should observe the client who has diabetes insipidus for signs of dehydration and hypovolemia. Decreased levels of antidiuretic hormone that may result from an injury to the hypothalamus will tend to cause marked diuresis and potential dehydration.**

1. Agitation and confabulation are not typical signs of diabetes insipidus. Typical signs of diabetes insipidus include polyuria and dehydration.

2. Clients who experience diabetes insipidus tend to present with dehydration due to polyuria, not fluid overload.

3. Hyperglycemia and metabolic acidosis are typical of diabetes mellitus, not diabetic insipidus.

Nursing Process: Implementing

Client Need: Health Promotion and Maintenance

7 - 2 7

① **The following equation can be used:**

To obtain 8 mg of meperidine:

$$\frac{50 \text{ mg}}{8 \text{ mg}} = \frac{1 \text{ cc}}{X}$$

50 X = 8 mg

X = 0.16 cc

To obtain 0.06 mg of atropine:

$$\frac{0.40 \text{ mg}}{0.06 \text{ mg}} = 0.15 \text{ cc}$$

2, 3, and 4. All are incorrect calculations.

Nursing Process: Implementing

Client Need: Physiological Integrity

7 - 2 8

④ **A rapid rise in the cerebrospinal fluid pressure while pressing on the neck veins indicates a normal finding. To assess for blockage in the vertebral canal, the Queckenstedt test (compression of the veins in the neck) is performed during a lumbar puncture procedure.**

1, 2, and 3. A blockage in the vertebral canal, presence of a tumor, or an infection such as meningitis will result in a minimal increase or no change in the cerebral spinal fluid pressure.

Nursing Process: Assessing

Client Need: Physiological Integrity

7 - 2 9

② **The goal of mobility within the limits imposed by the injury will be met when there is absence of contractures.**

1. Intact dry skin would meet the goal for the nursing diagnosis of "impairment of skin integrity related to sensory loss and immobility."

3. Seeks diversional activity would meet the goal for the nursing diagnosis of "ineffective individual coping related to impact of dysfunction on daily living."

4. Relaxed facial expression would meet the goal for the nursing diagnosis of "pain and discomfort related to treatment and prolonged immobility."

Nursing Process: Assessing
Client Need: Health Promotion and Maintenance

7 - 3 0

③ **The nurse will assign the client a score of 12 to 13. A score on the Glasgow Coma Scale (GCS) between 12 to 13 is a relatively high score indicating a relatively high level of consciousness.**

1. The Glasgow Coma Scale doesn't go as low as 1 to 2. The lowest score is a "1" for each of the 3 areas.

2. A score between 4 to 5 is very low, more appropriate for a client with no verbal response, abnormal flexion, and no eye opening.

4. The maximum score on the GCS is 15.

Nursing Process: Analyzing
Client Need: Health Promotion and Maintenance

7 - 3 1

② **The physician should be notified for the purpose of discussing a non-narcotic option for a client who has hypothyroidism and is in pain. Clients with hypothyroidism tend to have lower metabolic functioning. They are very susceptible to the effects of narcotics and have an increased risk of respiratory depression. It is prudent to avoid the use of narcotics in clients with acute hypothyroidism.**

1. This prescription should be verified since this client is at risk for respiratory depression due to hypothyroidism.

3. Analgesia should be administered for pain.

4. The route should not be altered in a medication prescription.

Nursing Process: Implementing
Client Need: Physiological Integrity

7 - 3 2

①　**Nursing assessment of the client's vision prior to surgery would reveal loss of visual acuity. Dense cataracts appear as gray opacity of the lens and impede the visual acuity of the eye.**

2.　Cataracts do not cause diplopia (double vision).

3.　Visual fatigue is not associated with cataracts.

4.　Floating filaments (floaters) are associated with retinal detachment, not cataracts.

Nursing Process: Analyzing

Client Need: Physiological Integrity

7 - 3 3

①　**Drowsiness is an early indication of increased intracranial pressure (ICP).**

2, 3, and 4.　Vomiting, hemiplegia, and widening pulse pressure are later signs of increased intracranial pressure.

Nursing Process: Analyzing

Client Need: Physiological Integrity

7 - 3 4

③　**The assessment technique that determines oculomotor nerve (CNIII) damage involves shining a penlight directly into the right eye and observing pupillary responses of both eyes. Direct and consensual pupillary responses should be observed. The lack of direct and consensual responses suggest oculomotor damage.**

1.　The ophthalmoscope is used for assessing the ocular media and for examination of the retina. However, this would not give any information about the oculomotor nerve.

2.　The Snellen chart assesses visual acuity but does not give information about the oculomotor nerve.

4.　Shining a penlight on the bridge of the nose and noting where the reflection is on each eye will assess the anterior chamber of the eye for normal transparency, not oculomotor damage.

Nursing Process: Assessing

Client Need: Physiological Integrity

7 - 3 5

③ **Pain behind the ear is indicative of mastoiditis, not otitis media.**

1, 2, and 4. Common behaviors of young children with otitis media include tugging at the earlobes and turning the head from side to side. Otitis media is not unusual in young children because their eustachian tubes are short, wide, and straight, characteristics that contribute to the spread of inflammation.

Nursing Process: Assessing
Client Need: Physiological Integrity

7 - 3 6

④ **The child with a brain tumor is most likely to have signs of increased intracranial pressure and problems with balance and coordination because most brain tumors in children are located in the cerebellum.**

1, 2, and 3. Abnormal results to pupil reflexes, deep tendon reflexes, and the number recall test are related to cranial nerves and memory. Most brain tumors in children are in the cerebellum and therefore cause increased intracranial pressure and problems with balance and coordination.

Nursing Process: Evaluating
Client Need: Physiological Integrity

7 - 3 7

② **The most likely assessment finding for a child admitted for a possible ventriculoperitoneal shunt revision would be diplopia. Strabismus (crossed eyes) and diplopia (double vision) may occur, not cranial enlargement. Signs of the condition are related to the increased intracranial pressure associated with hydrocephalus.**

1. The cranial sutures are closed in a 6-year-old. Therefore, the skull cannot enlarge to cause sunset eyes.

3. This is a "cracked pot" sound upon skull percussion when the skull is enlarged. This child is 6 years old and the cranial sutures are closed.

4. A high-pitched cry is most often associated with brain damage. There is no reason to believe that this child has brain damage.

Nursing Process: Assessing
Client Need: Health Promotion and Maintenance

7 - 3 8

④ **The most appropriate nursing diagnosis for a 15-month-old who has had a myelomeningocele repair would be altered growth and development, gross motor. At 15 months of age, a child is in a stage of active gross motor learning. Paralysis of the legs would interfere in this process.**

1. Fifteen months of age is too early for normal bladder continence.

2. Impaired verbal communication is not a problem with children who have had myelomeningocele repair.

3. Fifteen months of age is too early for normal bowel continence.

Nursing Process: Analyzing

Client Need: Physiological Integrity

7 - 3 9

① **The development of shock is characterized by a dropping blood pressure and a rising pulse rate. Therefore, a blood pressure of 100/60 and a pulse of 120 would signal shock in the client whose baseline blood pressure and pulse were 130/80 and 80.**

2. Signs of developing postoperative shock would include an increase in pulse rate, not a decrease. Also, the blood pressure would drop significantly.

3. Signs of developing postoperative shock would include a decrease in the blood pressure, not an increase.

4. Signs of developing postoperative shock would include a decrease in blood pressure, not an increase. Also, the pulse rate would increase, not decrease.

Nursing Process: Evaluating

Client Need: Physiological Integrity

7 - 4 0

② **An infant who has bacterial meningitis should have behavior monitored at each encounter. Meningitis is an inflammation of the meninges of the brain caused by bacteria or viruses. Behavior is a good indicator of intracranial pressure and is often an early sign of changes in intracranial pressure.**

1. Weight and head circumference should be assessed daily, not every 8 hours.

3. Kernig's sign (pain in the 3 hamstring muscles when attempting to extend the leg after flexing the thigh upon the abdomen) needs to be evaluated for initial diagnosis only.

4. Fontanels should be evaluated at least once every 8 hours. Evaluating fontanels only once in 24 hours would not be adequate due to the possibility of increased intracranial pressure.

Nursing Process: Implementing

Client Need: Physiological Integrity

7 - 4 1

(1) **Flushing the eyes with copious amounts of water is a first-aid measure and is very effective in reducing eye damage. Strong chemicals may injure the eyes. Removal of the hazardous chemical is the first priority.**

2 and 3. Neither sodium bicarbonate irrigation nor lidocaine ointment are indicated to treat chemical splashes to the eye.

4. Atropine solution is used to dilate the pupil for examination or procedure purposes.

Nursing Process: Implementing
Client Need: Physiological Integrity

7 - 4 2

(1) **Walking ability is the most appropriate assessment to perform on a preschool-age child who is suspected of having a brain tumor. Most brain tumors in children are in the cerebellum brain stem. Pressure on the cerebellum will affect its function of balance and coordination.**

2. The head will not enlarge in the preschool-age child in response to increased intracranial content since the cranium sutures are closed.

3. Circulation and oxygenation are not affected.

4. Vocabulary is a function of the cerebrum and most brain tumors in children are located in the cerebellum.

Nursing Process: Assessing
Client Need: Health Promotion and Maintenance

7 - 4 3

(4) **The purpose for a lumbar puncture in this situation is to test for the presence of blood. The presence of blood in the CSF indicates a cerebral bleed. Therefore, the initiation of heparin therapy may be based on these results.**

1. Elevation of intracranial pressure is usually treated with medications.

2. Although the cerebral spinal fluid (CSF) may be tested for many things, the purpose in this situation is to test for the presence of blood prior to the initiation of heparin therapy.

3. Administering heparin via lumbar puncture is inappropriate.

Nursing Process: Evaluating
Client Need: Health Promotion and Maintenance

7 - 4 4

  ① **The nurse should determine if the client has been exposed to chicken pox. The virus that caused herpes zoster appears to be identical to the causative agent of chicken pox.**

  2. Ulceration of the mouth and lips is not associated with the development of herpes zoster.

  3. A new shaving cream might be associated with contact dermatitis, not herpes zoster.

  4. Food allergies are not associated with herpes zoster.

Nursing Process: Assessing
Client Need: Physiological Integrity

7 - 4 5

  ① **Activities should be performed in the same order each day for clients experiencing organic brain syndrome. A stable, predictable environment is crucial in minimizing the confusion that comes with memory loss.**

2 and 4. Clients with organic brain syndrome have difficulty remembering recent events and new faces. It would be best to converse with the client about events and people that are remembered from the past.

  3. Providing a variety of activities for clients who have difficulty remembering recent events would not be helpful. It is likely to increase the client's confusion.

Nursing Process: Implementing
Client Need: Health Promotion and Maintenance

7 - 4 6

  ③ **Individuals who are experiencing right-sided homonymous hemianopsia should be taught to compensate by turning the head to the right. This will help minimize the deficit. When clients experience right-sided homonymous hemianopsia, they are unable to see out of the right side of each eye.**

Nursing Process: Implementing
Client Need: Health Promotion and Maintenance

7 - 4 7

③ **Clients who are scheduled for an electroencephalography (EEG) should be told not to drink fluids that contain caffeine, such as coffee and cola drinks. Caffeine is a central nervous system stimulant and could distort the electroencephalography results.**

1. Anticonvulsants, tranquilizers, barbiturates, and other sedatives such as diazepam (Valium) should be withheld for 24 to 48 hours (not 4 hours) prior to the EEG because they can alter the brain wave pattern.

2. There is no need to restrict food or fluids prior to an EEG unless they contain caffeine.

4. The nurse should explain the procedure and advise the client against consuming anything that contains caffeine.

Nursing Process: Implementing
Client Need: Health Promotion and Maintenance

7 - 4 8

③ **Encouraging deep breaths can help keep intracranial pressure down. Carbon dioxide (PaCO2) causes cerebral vasodilation and increases intracranial pressure. To lower carbon dioxide levels, the client should be encouraged to deep breathe. Hyperventilation lowers carbon dioxide levels.**

1 and 2. Keeping the head of the bed flat and placing a pillow under the knees increases intracranial pressure.

4. Administering 5% dextrose in water at 50 cc per hour will increase circulating fluid volume and thereby increase intracranial pressure.

Nursing Process: Implementing
Client Need: Physiological Integrity

7 - 4 9

② **One dose will contain 180 mg.**

1, 3, and 4. All are incorrect calculations.

Nursing Process: Implementing
Client Need: Physiological Integrity

7 - 5 0

① **A prescription for dipyridamole (Persantine) should be questioned for a client experiencing an acute hemorrhagic stroke. Dipyridamole (Persantine) is an antiplatelet agent that could promote further bleeding in the client with an acute hemorrhagic stroke.**

2, 3, and 4. Diazepam (Valium), phenytoin (Dilantin), and dexamethasone (Dexadron) are all appropriate medications to administer.

Nursing Process: Implementing
Client Need: Physiological Integrity

7 - 5 1

② **The nurse will anticipate related neurological deficits such as distension of the urinary bladder. Diminished sensation in the lower extremities following a motor vehicle accident is indicative of a neurological deficit related to spinal cord injury involving the lumbar and sacral regions.**

1, 3, and 4. Pupil size and reaction, respiratory distress, and the presence of a headache and nausea are signs of head injury unrelated to the presenting neurological symptom of decreased sensation in the lower extremities.

Nursing Process: Analyzing
Client Need: Physiological Integrity

7 - 5 2

① **Preoperative assessment of an infant prior to the surgical repair of a myelomeningocele should include ongoing fontanel status. Hydrocephalus is a common condition that may develop pre- or post-operatively with children who have a myelomeningocele. Ongoing fontanel assessment along with measurement of the head circumference would help monitor for hydrocephalus.**

2, 3, and 4. Hip dysplasia, bowel incontinence, and pain sensation below the defect are conditions that may be present at birth but do not need immediate attention and are not life threatening. Assessment does not need to be ongoing.

Nursing Process: Assessing
Client Need: Physiological Integrity

Practice Test 8

Renal System with Fluids and Electrolytes

8 - 1

Which of the following electrolyte imbalances is often associated with hypocalcemia?

1. hyperkalemia
2. hypoglycemia
3. hyperglycemia
4. hypomagnesemia

8 - 2

A 55-year-old female client has had frequent urinary tract infections. Which statement by the client indicates a need for further teaching?

1. "I will drink plenty of fluids."
2. "I will use bubble bath when bathing."
3. "I will wash my hands after going to the bathroom."
4. "I will wipe from the front to the back after passing a stool."

8 - 3

A 4-year-old child is being treated for a urinary tract infection. Ampicillin by mouth 4 times a day has been prescribed. The most appropriate teaching about this medication when prescribed for the treatment of a urinary tract infection is:

1. A full glass of water should be given with each dose.
2. Doses should be administered every 6 hours.
3. Chewable tablets are as effective as capsules and are easier for a child this age to take.
4. Allergy is more likely to occur when penicillin is given 4 times daily rather than twice daily.

8 - 4

A client with a long history of diabetes has developed chronic renal insufficiency secondary to diabetes. The physician has prescribed an 1800-Kcalorie renal diet. This diet consists of:

1. Kcalorie (1800) with sodium and potassium restriction.
2. sodium (1800 mg) with potassium restriction.
3. Kcalorie (1800) with 4 g sodium.
4. Kcalorie (1800) with 2 g sodium.

8 - 5

A client is scheduled for an intravenous pyelogram. Which of the following data would be most important for the nurse to know and record before this procedure is carried out?

1. urine negative for sugar and acetone
2. history of allergies
3. Has the client received a recent thyroid scan?
4. frequency of urination

8 - 6

A 33-year-old client is seen in the clinic and diagnosed with acute pyelonephritis. The client is placed on bed rest and given fluids ad lib. The client asks you why it is necessary to stay in bed. You will teach the client that bed rest will:

1. prevent respiratory infection by reducing the client's contact with other people.
2. ensure safety while the client has toxins in the bloodstream.
3. assist the client's body defenses in combating infection.
4. control ascending urinary infection by maintaining a horizontal position.

8 - 7

When teaching a client who is experiencing end-stage renal disease how to diminish the irritating effects of pruritus, the nurse will instruct the client to:

1. take frequent warm baths.
2. take tepid baths with emollients.
3. gently rub the skin with the palmar surface of the hands.
4. apply antihistamine cream to the skin every 8 hours.

8 - 8

A routine urinalysis was requested by the physician. To prevent contamination during the collection of the specimen, the nurse should:

1. wear gloves when handling the urine specimen.
2. wash hands before handling the specimen.
3. collect the specimen in a prelabeled container.
4. use sterile specimen containers only.

8 - 9

A client is receiving an intravenous infusion of D5W in 0.45% normal saline at 125 ml per hour through an infusion pump. Which of the following actions by a new graduate nurse needs further attention from the charge nurse?

1. ensuring that the volume infused coincides with the time tape on the intravenous bottle
2. adjusting the height of the pump attachment to ensure that the intravenous fluid flows by gravity
3. ensuring that the intravenous tubes are not pinched or kinked
4. including the infusion device used in the documentation of the intravenous therapy

8 - 1 0

A child with acute glomerulonephritis may experience all of the following manifestations. Which one indicates a possible complication?

1. hematuria
2. periorbital edema
3. headache
4. anorexia

8 - 1 1

A 2-year-old is in the acute phase of nephrotic syndrome. Which observation would be most important for the nurse to report to the child's health-care provider?

1. a cloudy nasal discharge
2. ate only a few bites of each meal yesterday
3. lethargic and easily fatigued
4. edema in the genital area

8 - 1 2

Your client is receiving a continuous infusion of the antineoplastic agent doxorubicin via a peripheral intravenous line. You observe a bleb at the infusion site of the client's intravenous infusion. Which of the following interventions will you take initially?

1. Lower the height of the infusion container.
2. Stop the fluid infusion.
3. Flush the infusion tubing with isotonic saline solution.
4. Slow the infusion rate.

8 - 1 3

A client is scheduled for an intravenous pyelography. Which of the following information is most important for the nurse to obtain from the client before this procedure?

1. a 24-hour urine output
2. thyroid functioning
3. history of allergies
4. adequacy of bowel evacuation

8 - 1 4

When developing a plan of care for an older client following a perineal prostatectomy, the nurse should include gradual supervised ambulation to:

1. shift the center of gravity in the body forward.
2. promote use of extensor rather than flexor muscles.
3. minimize the response to orthostatic reflex stimulation.
4. deter ossification of the long bones.

8 - 1 5

A client had a perineal prostatectomy. Because the client was in a lithotomy position for the operative procedure, the nurse will perform which of the following measures during the early postoperative period?

1. Turn the client from side to side and place a pillow between the legs.
2. Encourage flexion and extension exercises of the legs and apply elastic stocking.
3. Elevate the foot of the bed to 15 degrees and put a pillow at the head of the bed.
4. Place the head of the bed up and the feet down and put a pillow at the foot of the bed.

8 - 1 6

The nurse is teaching a client with an indwelling urinary catheter how to help prevent bladder infections. The nurse will plan to emphasize which of the following?

1. Encourage the client to eat the diet that is provided.
2. Have the client drink liberal amounts of fluid.
3. Tell the client to drink 1 glass of cranberry juice each day.
4. Instruct the client to keep the drainage bag level with the top of the mattress.

8 - 1 7

A client with the syndrome of inappropriate antidiuretic hormone is complaining of muscle cramps and weakness. The nurse will associate these complaints with:

1. hyponatremia.
2. hyperkalemia.
3. hyperchloremia.
4. hypercalcemia.

8 - 1 8

An adult client with cancer has an implanted venous access device. You are preparing to insert a specially designed needle to institute a prolonged continuous infusion of fluids. At what angle should you insert this needle?

1. 15 degrees
2. 30 degrees
3. 45 degrees
4. 90 degrees

8 - 1 9

During a hemodialysis, a client is receiving antibiotics. How can air be prevented from getting into the mechanical kidney?

1. Place the client with the head lower than the legs and feet.
2. Establish an intermittent infusion cap to administer the antibiotic.
3. Check the administration set every 5 minutes.
4. Aspirate all air from the intravenous bag prior to administration.

8 - 2 0

Following a transurethral resection of the prostate, a prescription for belladonna and opium suppositories for bladder spasms is to be administered. Which of the following historical information should alert the nurse for potential complications if belladonna and opium suppositories are administered?

1. history of peptic ulcers
2. seizure disorders with unknown causes
3. migraine headaches
4. glaucoma

8 - 2 1

The nurse is preparing a client for an abdominal paracentesis. It is essential for the nurse to take which of the following actions?

1. Instruct the client about how to participate in the procedure.
2. Withhold oral intake for at least 24 hours before the procedure.
3. Have the client empty the bladder immediately prior to the procedure.
4. Provide the client with a rolled blanket to place against the back to maintain a sitting position during the procedure.

8 - 2 2

A client's intravenous fluids contain potassium chloride to replace potassium lost during gastric suctioning. The nurse will observe the client for symptoms of potassium deficiency that include:

1. abdominal muscle spasticity.
2. labored respirations.
3. leg muscle weakness.
4. hypertension.

8 - 2 3

An 82-year-old client is admitted to the hospital with benign prostatic hypertrophy. Which of the following questions would be appropriate for the nurse to ask when assessing the client's symptoms?

1. "Do you have difficulty in voiding?"
2. "Is there a discharge from your penis?"
3. "Is there swelling in your groin?"
4. "Do you have tenderness in your scrotum?"

8 - 2 4

A 46-year-old is admitted to the hospital with a diagnosis of renal calculi. Which of the following actions would be most important for the nurse to initiate for the client?

1. Provide a quiet environment.
2. Strain all urine.
3. Tell the client not to eat or drink anything.
4. Advise the client to remain in bed.

8 - 2 5

A client who has been scheduled for dialysis has a blood urea nitrogen of 63 mg/dL, a creatinine of 4.5 mg/dL, and a potassium of 7.4 mEq/L. A kayexelate enema is prescribed. You know the purpose of the enema is to:

1. empty the bowel prior to the dialysis.
2. lower the blood urea nitrogen.
3. lower the potassium level.
4. increase the creatinine.

8 - 2 6

Which of the following microorganisms is responsible for the majority of urinary tract infections in female clients?

1. *Escherichia coli*
2. *Nesseria gonorrhea*
3. *Corpus albicans*
4. *Haemophilus influenzae*

8 - 2 7

Your client has had a nephrectomy for removal of a Wilms' tumor. The least appropriate nursing intervention for a child who has had a nephrectomy for removal of a Wilms' tumor is:

1. monitoring urine for gross and microscopic hematuria.
2. monitoring bowel sounds and abdominal distention.
3. monitoring vital signs, including blood pressure.
4. encouraging deep breathing and coughing often.

8 - 2 8

A client has developed an acute renal insufficiency following antibiotic therapy. Dopamine intravenous infusion was prescribed to restore renal function. The mechanism of dopamine's therapeutic action includes:

1. increasing renal function.
2. lowering blood pressure.
3. increasing cardiac output.
4. decreasing serum potassium levels.

8 - 2 9

An infant who is on intake and output measurements spits up all over the bib and nightgown. Which action should be indicated?

1. Caution the parents to be more observant and catch all emesis in a basin.
2. Weigh the soiled items before and after laundering to estimate fluid loss.
3. Suggest that the parents call for assistance the next time vomiting occurs.
4. Provide a bath basin to catch any emesis.

8 - 3 0

A client with chronic obstructive pulmonary disease developed a respiratory infection that was successfully treated with gentamicin sulfate. The client is now complaining of nausea and anorexia. Blood work reveals a potassium of 4.8 mmol/L, blood urea nitrogen of 36 mg/dL, creatinine of 3.2 mg/dL, sodium of 148 mEq/L, and a glucose of 116 mg/dL. Which problem is suggested by these results?

1. acute renal failure
2. hypokalemia
3. dehydration
4. hypoglycemia

8 - 3 1

A client is to receive 1000 cc of D5W over a 6-hour period. The drop factor on the infusion set is 15. The nurse will infuse the fluids at:

1. 16 gtts per minute.
2. 28 gtts per minute.
3. 41 gtts per minute.
4. 160 gtts per minute.

8 - 3 2

A client is admitted with a provisional diagnosis of benign prostatic hypertrophy. To assist in assessing urinary status, the physician writes a prescription to "catheterize for residual urine." To administer this prescription, the nurse should explain the procedure and:

1. insert an indwelling urinary catheter, record 24-hour output, then remove the indwelling catheter.
2. ask the client to void, insert a straight catheter, drain the bladder and measure output, and remove the catheter and record.
3. insert an indwelling urinary catheter, drain the bladder, instill 500 cc of sterile saline into the bladder, and ask the client to void.
4. ask the client to void, insert a straight catheter, instill methylene blue solution into the bladder, and have the client void and record.

8 - 3 3

A client is experiencing acute renal failure that is postrenal in nature. You know that this is probably due to:

1. hypovolemia.
2. cardiogenic shock.
3. nephrotoxic substances.
4. urethral obstruction.

8 - 3 4

Your client is experiencing dependent edema and has been receiving furosemide 20 mg intravenously bid for the past 3 days. An appropriate nursing intervention would be to:

1. encourage po fluid intake.
2. keep the room dimly lit.
3. monitor electrolytes.
4. avoid and discourage high potassium.

8 - 3 5

A client is scheduled for a nephrectomy. You will plan to give the client's preoperative medication:

1. prior to morning care to allow for observations of the client's reaction to the medication.
2. prior to morning care to promote optimal relaxation for the client.
3. after morning care to prevent disturbing the client until surgery.
4. after morning care because the medication would otherwise interfere with the care.

8 - 3 6

A client has a vulvectomy and returns to her room with an indwelling urethral catheter attached to a gravity drainage and a perineal dressing held in place with a T-binder. When performing an initial postoperative assessment, the nurse will expect the urine to appear:

1. bright red.
2. cloudy.
3. blood-tinged.
4. amber.

8 - 3 7

A client has just returned from a cystoscopy. An essential nursing intervention at this time would be to:

1. assess the color of the client's urine.
2. keep the client npo for 2 hours.
3. assess the client's gag reflex prior to feeding.
4. encourage the client to ambulate immediately following the examination.

8 - 3 8

A client is to receive 1500 ml of 5% dextrose in water over a period of 8 hours. The drop factor is 20 gtts/ml. The fluid should infuse at which of the following rates?

1. 43 gtts per minute
2. 52 gtts per minute
3. 63 gtts per minute
4. 72 gtts per minute

8 - 3 9

Your client had a cystectomy for the purpose of removing a large tumor in the urinary bladder. An ileal conduit was performed. You know to record the client's urinary volume:

1. every hour.
2. every 30 minutes.
3. at each shift change.
4. every 2 hours.

8 - 4 0

Your client is receiving cortisone acetate 100 mg po and hydrochlorothiazide 50 mg po daily. You will monitor which of the following laboratory values?

1. elevated serum potassium
2. low serum potassium
3. low hemoglobin
4. low serum glucose

8 - 4 1

With which of the following conditions is dehydration least likely to occur?

1. pneumonia
2. meningitis
3. nephrotic syndrome
4. elevated blood sugar

8 - 4 2

After a transurethral prostatectomy, your client is returned to your unit from recovery. The client has an indwelling urethral catheter and is receiving continuous bladder irrigations with normal saline solution. When monitoring the irrigation, you should:

1. clamp the flow from the irritating solution for the specified time, then open to allow a designated amount of solution to flush the bladder.
2. infuse no more than 50 ml of irrigating solution, then apply a moderate amount of suction to withdraw the solution.
3. check to be sure that the solution outflow corresponds to the irrigation inflow and patency of the catheter is maintained.
4. warm the irrigating solution to body temperature and infuse at 100 cc per hour.

8 - 4 3

Your client is in renal failure and is being treated with hemodialysis. Because of an infected fistula, the decision has been made to initiate peritoneal dialysis. You explain to your client that this procedure:

1. requires the injection of dialysate into the digestive tract and allows electrolyte exchange to occur there.

2. may only be used for a maximum of 2 exchanges.

3. utilizes the peritoneum as the semipermeable membrane.

4. is much quicker in resolving electrolyte balance than hemodialysis.

8 - 4 4

Sodium polystyrene sulfonate is prescribed for a client. When administering this medication, the nurse will expect the desired therapeutic effect to occur through which of the following actions?

1. shifts in intracellular potassium

2. decreased potassium intoxication

3. lower serum sodium levels

4. increased serum sulfate levels

8 - 4 5

Your client has received intravenous fluids for 3 days postoperatively. You plan to observe for any signs of fluid overload. You know that signs of fluid overload include:

1. weight loss.

2. decrease in blood pressure.

3. depressed inspiration rate.

4. coughing and wheezing.

8 - 4 6

A client enters the hospital in acute renal failure. The client complains of drowsiness and nausea and has Kussmaul breathing. Laboratory tests indicate a serum potassium of 6.8 mEq/liter, serum 120 mEq/liter, and a blood pH of 7.2. Which prescription should be questioned?

1. polystyrene sodium sulfonate 50 gm per rectum, as enema

2. a 2000-calorie, high-carbohydrate, high-protein diet when nausea subsides

3. hypertonic glucose (25%), 300 cc with 35 units of Regular insulin per intravenous infusion over 1 hour

4. limit po fluids per 8 hours to no more than 100 cc above the urinary output for the previous 8 hours

8 - 4 7

Which of the following information about nephrolithiasis would be accurate?

1. The incidence of nephrolithiasis is greater in women than in men.
2. The incidence of nephrolithiasis is greatest in the African American population.
3. Low urine volume will increase the risk of nephrolithiasis.
4. Nephrolithiasis will cause constant, aching pain.

8 - 4 8

Following a transurethral resection of the prostate, you perform an initial assessment and find vital signs stable; client alert and complaining of feeling a need to void; a 3-way #24 indwelling catheter with continuous normal saline irrigation draining well; and catheter drainage pinkish-red with numerous tiny clots. Your first action will be to:

1. notify the physician of the urine color and the passage of clots.
2. palpate the suprapubic area gently for signs of bladder fullness.
3. position and anchor the catheter by taping it to lie horizontally across the upper thigh.
4. encourage the client to bear down slightly as if trying to void in order to interrupt nerve impulses from the irritated internal bladder sphincter.

Practice Test 8

Answers, Rationales, and Explanations

8 - 1

④ Hypocalcemia is often associated with the electrolyte imbalance of hypomagnesemia. Magnesium is one of the electrolytes that affects the parathyroid hormone levels. Low magnesium levels therefore have the tendency to lower calcium levels, too, since parathyroid hormone (PTH) directly affects serum calcium levels. An increase in serum magnesium will often cause a corresponding rise in serum calcium level.

1, 2, and 3. Neither serum potassium levels nor serum glucose levels directly influence serum calcium levels, unlike the association between magnesium and the parathyroid hormone.

Nursing Process: Evaluating
Client Need: Physiological Integrity

8 - 2

② A woman with a urinary tract infection should be taught not to use bubble bath when bathing. Inflammation of the bladder and ureters can develop from exposure to ingredients contained in bubble baths and shampoos.

1, 3, and 4. Urinary tract infections can be treated and prevented by drinking plenty of water, washing the hands, and wiping from the front to the back after passing a stool.

Nursing Process: Analyzing
Client Need: Physiological Integrity

8 - 3

② The most appropriate teaching about ampicillin when prescribed for the treatment of urinary tract infection is to administer the dosage every 6 hours. Administering ampicillin every 6 hours will assure a uniform high blood level of the drug. Maintaining a steady high blood level is necessary for effective treatment.

1. Fluids need to be given frequently, not just when administering the medication.
3. Ampicillin is not available in chewable tablets.
4. Allergy can occur at any time and dosing frequency does not contribute to allergy.

Nursing Process: Implementing
Client Need: Health Promotion and Maintenance

8 - 4

1. **An 1800-Kcalorie renal diet consists of 1800 Kcal for calorie control, 2 g sodium, and restricted potassium for management of renal failure.**

2. The Kcalories should be 1800, sodium should be 2 g rather than 1800 mg, and the potassium restriction is not specified.

3. The diet should contain 1800 Kcalories and 2 g of sodium with potassium restriction.

4. This diet is inappropriate for sodium and potassium because of renal impairment.

Nursing Process: Implementing
Client Need: Health Promotion and Maintenance

8 - 5

2. **A client should be assessed for a history of allergies before having an intravenous pyelogram. Intravenous pyelogram (IVP) requires an iodine radiopaque dye. The client may have an allergy to iodine and may therefore be allergic to the IVP dye. Clients are given a clear liquid diet on the evening before the procedure, since food in the stomach could obstruct the view of the urinary structure. The client is given only water until bedtime, then npo for 8 to 10 hours before the test. Usually, laxatives are given the night before and an enema until clear in the morning before the test. The nurse should record the client's reaction to the dye such as tingling, numbness, and palpitations. After the procedure, fluids are forced to remove the dye and relieve any dehydration.**

1. It is not necessary that the urine be negative for sugar and acetone in order for the client to have an IVP.

3. A recent thyroid scan would not interfere with an IVP. However, the reverse is not true. A recent IVP could interfere with the results of a thyroid scan.

4. Frequency of urination would not affect the results of an IVP.

Nursing Process: Assessing
Client Need: Safe, Effective Care Environment

8 - 6

③ **Clients experiencing pyelonephritis (inflammation of the kidney) are placed on bed rest because bed rest will assist the body's defenses in combating infection by conserving energy and allowing the body to use its resources to combat infection.**

1 and 2. This client has pyelonephritis. Bed rest will neither prevent respiratory infections nor ensure safety while there are toxins in the body. Bed rest will, however, help the body to combat infection in the kidneys.

4. Maintaining a horizontal position would worsen pyelonephritis by allowing bacterial infection to travel upward to the pelvis of the kidney (pyelonephritis results from the spread of infection from the lower urinary tract).

Nursing Process: Implementing

Client Need: Health Promotion and Maintenance

8 - 7

② **Clients with end-stage renal disease (ESRD) may have pruritus (severe itching of the skin). Tepid baths with emollients are soothing and remove the bile salts that exude onto the surface of the skin.**

1. Warm baths will cause further drying of the skin and contribute to pruritus.

3. Rubbing the skin may cause further skin irritation.

4. Creams are used as an adjunct but they are costly.

Nursing Process: Implementing

Client Need: Physiological Integrity

8 - 8

① **To prevent contamination during the collection of a urine specimen, the nurse should wear gloves when handling the specimen. Wearing gloves will prevent contamination of the specimen and the collector. This meets the requirements of the Occupational Safety and Health Administration (OSHA).**

2. The nurse should wear gloves.

3. It is not necessary that the specimen container be prelabeled as long as the nurse wears gloves when handling the specimen.

4. It is not necessary to use a sterile container when collecting a routine urine specimen for urinalysis.

Nursing Process: Planning

Client Need: Safe, Effective Care Environment

8 - 9

② A new graduate is in need of attention from the charge nurse if the graduate adjusts the height of the pump attachment. It is not necessary to adjust the height of the pump attachment to ensure that the intravenous fluid flows by gravity. Infusion pumps do not depend on gravity pressure; they can be placed at any level. Eye contact is convenient for checking its functioning.

1. The volume infused should coincide with the time tape on the intravenous bottle.
3. The intravenous tube should not be pinched or kinked.
4. Documentation should include the device used to infuse the fluids.

Nursing Process: Implementing
Client Need: Health Promotion and Maintenance

8 - 1 0

③ A possible complication associated with acute glomerulonephritis would be a headache. Headache may be an indicator of encephalopathy due to hypertension. Other key indicators include dizziness, abdominal discomfort, and vomiting. Grand mal seizures may also occur. The most common cause of acute glomerulonephritis is a previous infection by group A beta-hemolytic streptococcus.

1. Hematuria (blood in the urine) is a clinical manifestation of glomerulonephritis, not a complication. The presence of hematuria is essential for a diagnosis of glomerulonephritis. The degree of hematuria may range from severe to microscopic. The color of the client's urine may be dark "tea-colored."
2. Edema is a clinical manifestation of glomerulonephritis, especially around the eyelids (periorbital) and in the ankles.
4. Nausea and vomiting are clinical manifestations of glomerulonephritis, not complications.

Nursing Process: Analyzing
Client Need: Physiological Integrity

8 - 1 1

① A cloudy nasal discharge from a child in the acute phase of nephrotic syndrome should be reported immediately to the child's health-care provider. A cloudy nasal discharge is an indicator of infection. Children with nephrotic syndrome (a kidney disorder manifested by proteinuria, hypoalbuminemia, and edema) are very susceptible to infection because of treatment with corticosteroids, loss of proteins, and generalized edema. Prompt treatment of infection is essential.

2, 3, and 4. Anorexia, lethargy, fatigue, and generalized edema are to be expected in this condition.

Nursing Process: Analyzing
Client Need: Health Promotion and Maintenance

8 - 1 2

② **The nurse should stop an intravenous fluid infusion immediately if extravasation (the escape of fluids into the surrounding tissues) is suspected. Doxorubicin (Adriamycin) is a vesicant (caustic, blister-forming medication) when it escapes from the vein into surrounding tissues.**

1, 3, and 4. The fluid should be stopped and the physician notified before any additional intervention is implemented.

Nursing Process: Implementing
Client Need: Safe, Effective Care Environment

8 - 1 3

③ **The information the nurse should obtain before scheduling an intravenous pyelography (IVP) is a history of allergies. An iodine-based radiopaque dye is used to perform an IVP. Clients with a history of allergy to iodine-based compounds or seafood are often allergic to the dye.**

1. The clients' 24-hour urine output will not affect IVP results.
2. A thyroid function evaluation will not affect IVP results.
4. Bowel evacuation is not a consideration when scheduling an IVP.

Nursing Process: Evaluating
Client Need: Safe, Effective Care Environment

8 - 1 4

③ **The nurse can minimize the older client's response to orthostatic reflex stimulation by supervised gradual ambulation. Postoperatively, older adults are more susceptible to orthostatic hypotension due to a decrease in the sensitivity of their baroreceptors to position change.**

1. The center of gravity affects balance but does not affect orthostatic hypotension.
2. Promoting the use of extensor rather than flexor muscles is helpful when treating and preventing contractures. However, this will not affect orthostatic hypotension.
4. Gradual supervision of ambulation does not deter ossification of long bones.

Nursing Process: Planning
Client Need: Physiological Integrity

8 - 1 5

② The nurse will encourage clients who have assumed a lithotomy position to flex and extend their legs. Also, elastic stockings may be applied. The lithotomy position (client lying on back with feet in stirrups, the hips acutely flexed and the thighs separated) places the client at increased risk for deep vein thrombosis. Encouraging flexion and extension exercises of the client's legs and applying elastic stockings will prevent venous stasis and thrombophlebitis.

1. Placing a pillow between the legs would be uncomfortable for a client who has had a perineal prostatectomy and would not prevent venous stasis and thrombophlebitis.

3. Elevating the head of the bed 15 degrees is not as effective in preventing venous stasis and thrombophlebitis as flexion and extension exercises of the legs along with elastic stockings.

4. Clients may be placed with the head of the bed up and the feet down to treat increased intracranial pressure. This client does not require such a position.

Nursing Process: Implementing
Client Need: Safe, Effective Care Environment

8 - 1 6

② The nurse will encourage the client who has an indwelling urinary catheter to drink liberal amounts of fluid. A high fluid intake will dilute the urine and decrease mucosal irritation. The increase in urine volume also facilitates maintenance of catheter patency.

1. Encouraging a well-balanced diet helps to maintain general good health. However, a specific action that should be encouraged to prevent infections associated with indwelling catheters is to consume liberal amounts of fluids.

3. One glass of cranberry juice will not provide enough consistent acidity to prevent urinary infections.

4. The drainage bag should be kept below the level of the client's bladder to prevent a backflow of contaminated urine into the client's bladder from the bag.

Nursing Process: Planning
Client Need: Physiological Integrity

8 - 1 7

① **The nurse will associate muscle cramps and weakness with hyponatremia. Hyponatremia (serum sodium below 135 mEq/liter) will cause muscle cramps and weakness in clients experiencing syndrome of inappropriate antidiuretic hormone (SIDH). These clients have a low urinary output with high specific gravity, a sudden weight gain, or a serum sodium decline. Excess antidiuretic hormone increases renal tubular permeability and the reabsorption of water into the circulation. This results in extracellular fluid expansion, followed by plasma osmolarity and serum sodium decline. Lastly, glomerular filtration rate rises and sodium levels decline.**

2. Hyperkalemia (serum potassium levels above 5.5 mg/dL) is not associated with SIDH. Signs of hyperkalemia include muscle weakness and impaired muscle functions, tremors, twitching, cardiac dysrhythmias, and cardiac arrest. Disease process associated with hyperkalemia includes Addison's disease and renal failure.

3. Hyperchloremia (serum chloride levels above 390 mg/dL) is not associated with SIDH. Signs of hyperchloremia include developing stupor, rapid deep breathing, and weakness that may lead to coma.

4. Hypercalcemia (serum calcium levels above 10.1 mg/dL) is not associated with SIDH. Signs of hypercalcemia include bone pain, flank pain due to renal calculi, and muscle hypotonicity.

Nursing Process: Analyzing
Client Need: Physiological Integrity

8 - 1 8

④ **For prolonged continuous infusions of fluids or chemotherapy, a 90-degree angled, specially-designed needle (Huber needle) is used for top entry ports. Straight Huber needles are available for bolus injections and blood withdrawn from both top- and side-entry ports. The angled bevel design of the Huber needle prevents coring of the rubber septum of the port and permits repeated insertion. A dressing is applied over the 90-degree needle to secure the needle position and prevent infection.**

1, 2, and 3. All are incorrect angles.

Nursing Process: Implementing
Client Need: Physiological Integrity

8 - 1 9

④ **The nurse will aspirate all the air from the intravenous bag. Aspirating all air from the intravenous bag creates a vacuum, disallowing air from entering the mechanical kidney.**

1. Placing the client in the Trendelenburg position (head lower than the legs and feet) will not prevent air from entering the machine.
2. It is not necessary to establish an intermittent infusion cap.
3. Checking the administration set every 5 minutes is not realistic.

Nursing Process: Planning
Client Need: Safe, Effective Care Environment

8 - 2 0

④ **A client with a history of glaucoma would be at risk for complications should belladonna and opium suppositories be administered. Belladonna and opium (B&O) suppositories are anticholinergic agents. These agents are contraindicated for clients with glaucoma because they impair outflow of aqueous humor and cause increased intraocular pressure. An acute attack of glaucoma could occur following the administration of an anticholinergic drug.**

1. A history of peptic ulcers would not interfere with the administration of B&O suppositories.
2. Clients with seizure disorders are not prohibited from taking B&O suppositories.
3. Clients who have a history of migraine headaches are not prohibited from taking B&O suppositories.

Nursing Process: Assessing
Client Need: Health Promotion and Maintenance

8 - 2 1

③ **It is essential that the nurse have the client empty the bladder immediately before an abdominal paracentesis. Having the client void will lessen the danger of accidentally piercing the bladder when the surgeon introduces the trocar through a stab wound below the umbilicus.**

1. The nurse should inform all clients about what is expected of them during any procedure, not just an abdominal paracentesis.
2. It is not necessary to withhold oral intake prior to an abdominal paracentesis.
4. The client can either remain in bed in an upright position (90 degress) or sit in a chair with a supportive back. It is not necessary to place a rolled blanket against the client's back.

Nursing Process: Planning
Client Need: Safe, Effective Care Environment

8 - 2 2

③ **Potassium depletion (hypokalemia) results in decreased muscular function which is manifested by weakness, flaccid paralysis, shallow respirations, decreased intestinal motility, abdominal distension, paralytic ileus, and vomiting. Other signs include decreased neuromuscular irritability and cardiac dysrhythmia.**

1. Abdominal muscle spasticity is not associated with potassium depletion. However, abdominal distension may be experienced.

2. In severe cases of hypokalemia, shallow respirations and respiratory paralysis may occur, not labored breathing.

4. Hypotension, not hypertension, may occur with potassium depletion.

Nursing Process: Analyzing
Client Need: Physiological Integrity

8 - 2 3

① **It would be appropriate for the nurse to ask if the client is experiencing difficulty voiding. As the prostate gland enlarges, it puts pressure on the urethra and causes urinary stasis, recurring infections, frequent urination, nocturia, and dysuria.**

2. A discharge from the penis is not associated with benign prostatic hypertrophy. However, discharge from the penis does occur with sexually transmitted diseases (STDs) such as gonorrhea.

3. Swelling in the groin is not associated with benign prostatic hypertrophy. However, swelling in the groin may be seen in conditions such as inguinal hernia.

4. Tenderness in the scrotum is associated with conditions such as testicular torsion.

Nursing Process: Assessing
Client Need: Safe, Effective Care Environment

8 - 2 4

② **All urine of a client suspected of having a renal or ureteral calculus should be strained in the event the stone is passed. Fluids are encouraged to assist stones in their downward passage and ambulation utilizes gravity in moving stones along.**

1. A quiet environment is not as important as straining all the client's urine for inspection of renal stones.

3. Food and fluids are not restricted. In fact, fluids are encouraged in an attempt to flush out the calculus.

4. Clients with renal or ureteral calculi may assume any position they wish. They do not need to remain in bed. Ambulation may actually help the calculus to pass.

Nursing Process: Implementing
Client Need: Physiological Integrity

8 - 2 5

③ **A sodium polystyrene sulfonate (Kayexalate) enema is administered to lower the client's potassium. Kayexalate is an electrolyte modifier that exchanges sodium ions for potassium in the intestines. The normal serum potassium is 3.5 to 5.5 mEq/L. A serum potassium level above 5.5 mEq/L is considered hyperkalemia and requires treatment.**

1. The Kayexalate enema may empty the bowel. However, emptying the bowel is not the intended effect of the Kayexalate.

2. The normal blood urea nitrogen (BUN) value ranges from 8 to 20 mg/dL. A BUN of 63 mg/dL is abnormally high and suggests renal disease. Obtaining a BUN level also aids in the assessment of dehydration. A Kayexalate enema will have little if any effect on a client's BUN level.

4. A normal creatinine level is 0.7 to 1.5 mg/dL. However, even though the client has a high creatinine level of 4.5 mg/dL, a Kayexalate enema would not have any effect on creatinine.

Nursing Process: Evaluating
Client Need: Physiological Integrity

8 - 2 6

① *Escherichia coli* **(E. coli) is the bacteria that is a normal part of the intestinal flora and is responsible for the majority of urinary tract infections in the female. Because of the proximity of the urethra to the rectum, women are more prone to urinary tract infections caused by this bacteria. Over 80% of urinary tract infections in women are caused by E. coli.**

2 and 3. *Nesseria gonorrhea* (N. gonorrhea) and *Corpus albicans* (C. albicans) typically produce vaginitis.

4. *Haemophilus influenzae* (H. influenzae) is associated with infections of the respiratory tract and ear.

Nursing Process: Evaluating
Client Need: Physiological Integrity

8 - 2 7

(1) The least appropriate nursing intervention for a child who has had a nephrectomy for the removal of a Wilms' tumor is monitoring urine for gross and microscopic hematuria. The affected kidney has been removed. Therefore, hematuria should not be present. The remaining kidney is left intact and undisturbed. A large transabdominal incision is made to allow for easy removal of the involved kidney (and adjacent adrenal gland) and visualization of the uninvolved kidney. Follow-up includes radiation and chemo-therapy with actinomycin D and vincristine.

2 and 3. In addition to the effects of general anesthesia, this client may develop adynamic ileus from the vincristine, edema in the abdomen from the radiation, and possible infections.

4.   The high and extensive abdominal incision contributes to a greater possibility of developing respiratory infections.

Nursing Process: Assessing
Client Need: Health Promotion and Maintenance

8 - 2 8

(1) Dopamine's therapeutic action includes increasing renal function. Dopamine hydrochloride (Intropin) affects both the alpha and beta adrenergic receptors of the sympathetic nervous system. At low doses (1 to 2 mg/kg/min), dopamine has a vasodilatory effect on the brain, kidneys, and other organs, thereby increasing renal perfusion and subsequent urinary output.

2.   With improved renal function, blood pressure will return to normal as an indirect action of the Intropin.

3.   Intropin does not directly improve cardiac output.

4.   With improved renal function, water and electrolyte excretions will increase; however, it is not the primary action of Intropin.

Nursing Process: Evaluating
Client Need: Physiological Integrity

8 - 2 9

(2) The nurse should weigh the soiled linens before and after laundering. Infants can dehydrate quickly since their bodies are composed of approximately 80% water.

1 and 3. It may not be possible for the nurse or the client's parents to account for all emesis by collecting it in a basin. Therefore, soiled bibs and nightgowns should be weighed before and after laundering.

4.   Even if the proper basins are available, vomiting may be sudden and unexpected and therefore not likely to be collected.

Nursing Process: Implementing
Client Need: Health Promotion and Maintenance

8 - 3 0

1. **The combination of a blood urea nitrogen (BUN) of 36 mg/dL (normal is 8 to 20 mg/dL) and a creatinine of 3.2 mg/dL (normal is 0.7 to 1.5 mg/dL) suggests renal failure. Renal failure occurs with gentamicin therapy because it is nephrotoxic.**

2 and 4. The client's serum potassium is within the normal range of 3.5 to 5.5 mmol/L as is the glucose whose normal range is 60 to 120 mg/dL.

3. Dehydration is often indicated by an elevated BUN but a normal creatinine.

Nursing Process: Analyzing
Client Need: Physiological Integrity

8 - 3 1

③ **Formula:**

$$\frac{\text{amount} \times \text{drop factor}}{\text{time (in minutes)}} = \frac{1,000 \times 15}{6 \times 60} = \frac{15,000}{360} = 41 \text{ drops per minute (41 gtts/min)}.$$

1, 2, and 4. All are incorrect calculations.

Nursing Process: Planning
Client Need: Safe, Effective Care Environment

8 - 3 2

② **Urine remaining in the bladder after voiding is called "residual urine." The amount is usually determined by catheterizing the client immediately after voiding. With normal or near-normal bladder functioning, the volume of residual urine is 50 cc or less. An indwelling urinary catheter may be used if a large amount of residual urine is expected and the physician has indicated that an indwelling catheter is to be left in place if a specified volume of residual urine is exceeded.**

1. Recording a 24-hour urine output is not the process one would follow to determine residual urine.

3. Placing sterile saline in the bladder may be initiated following a prostatectomy to relieve any obstruction that may cause discomfort. However, a sterile saline irrigation is not associated with the procedure for collecting residual urine.

4. Methylene blue helps to delineate the cause of a fistula. It is not associated with the procedure for collecting residual urine.

Nursing Process: Implementing
Client Need: Health Promotion and Maintenance

8 - 3 3

④ **Urethral obstruction is a typical cause of postrenal failure. Urethral obstruction causes urine to back up and pressure in the kidneys to rise. Postrenal failure refers to any condition occurring below the level of the kidney.**

1 and 2. Hypovolemic and cardiogenic shock may cause prerenal failure. Both cause systemic hypoperfusion and thus renal hypoperfusion.

3. Nephrotoxic substances (substances that damage kidney tissues) directly assault the nephron.

Nursing Process: Assessing
Client Need: Physiological Integrity

8 - 3 4

③ **Clients receiving furosemide should monitor electrolytes. Potassium and sodium are excreted in the urine of clients receiving furosemide (Lasix). Therefore, fluids and electrolytes should be monitored carefully in clients experiencing dependent edema.**

1. Encouraging fluids would be contraindicated for clients receiving diuretics.

2. Photosensitivity is not a common side effect of furosemide. There is no reason to keep the client's room dimly lit.

4. Persons on loop diuretics such as Lasix are at risk for hypokalemia. Therefore, you would encourage foods high in potassium.

Nursing Process: Implementing
Client Need: Health Promotion and Maintenance.

8 - 3 5

③ **The purpose of a preoperative medication is to relax the client, alleviate anxiety, and permit a smooth induction of anesthesia prior to surgery. Therefore, to prevent disturbing the client, the morning care should be completed before the preoperative medication is given.**

1 and 2. The preoperative medication is given to relax the client, allay anxiety, and permit a smooth induction of anesthesia. The client should not be disturbed after preoperative medication is given.

4. The preoperative medication is given after morning care not because it would interfere with the care. It is given after morning care so that the client will not be disturbed while the medication takes effect.

Nursing Process: Planning
Client Need: Safe, Effective Care Environment

8 - 3 6

④ **Following a vulvectomy, the initial postoperative assessment of the urine from the indwelling catheter should be amber (the normal color).**

1. A bright red color of urine would indicate possible hemorrhage and a complication of surgery.

2. Initially, a cloudy color would not be expected postoperatively because this would indicate an infection that would take time to develop.

3. Blood-tinged urine would indicate possible hemorrhage and a complication of surgery.

Nursing Process: Assessing
Client Need: Physiological Integrity

8 - 3 7

① **An essential nursing intervention at this time would be to observe the client's urine to see if it is bloody or cloudy. A cystoscopy is a procedure in which the physician views the interior of the bladder and urethra with a cystoscope.**

2. The client should be encouraged to drink plenty of fluids. Intake and output should be monitored.

3. The gag reflex does not need to be assessed because the client's throat has not been anesthetized.

4. The client is usually kept on bed rest for the first 4 to 6 hours after the procedure.

Nursing Process: Implementing
Client Need: Physiological Integrity

8 - 3 8

③ **The fluid should infuse at 63 drops per minute.**

$$\frac{\text{amount} \times \text{drop factor}}{\text{time (in minutes)}} = \frac{1,500 \times 20}{8 \times 60} = \frac{30,000}{480} = 63 \text{ gtts/min}).$$

1, 2, and 4. All are incorrect calculations.

Nursing Process: Implementing
Client Need: Safe, Effective Care Environment

8 - 3 9

① **The postoperative urinary volume should be checked every hour. The kidneys normally produce a minimum of 30 cc of urine every hour. A minimum of 240 cc for an 8-hour period is expected.**

2. Every 30 minutes is too soon to make a correct evaluation since the kidneys normally produce a minimum of 30 cc of urine every hour.

3 and 4. Checking the urinary volume at each shift change or every 2 hours does not give an accurate recording of the urine being excreted every hour.

Nursing Process: Implementing
Client Need: Health Promotion and Maintenance

8 - 4 0

② **The nurse will monitor closely for low serum potassium. Concurrent use of a thiazide diuretic such as hydrochlorothiazide (Ezide) may increase the potassium-wasting effect of cortisone acetate. Therefore, the client should be monitored for low serum potassium.**

1. Concurrent use of these medications will tend to lower, not elevate, the serum potassium level.

3. Cortisone acetate and hydrochlorothiazide does not affect hemoglobin.

4. Serum glucose tends to be higher than normal, not lower, while a client is on cortisone acetate.

Nursing Process: Planning
Client Need: Physiological Integrity

8 - 4 1

③ **Dehydration is least likely to occur among clients who have nephrotic syndrome.**

1. Fluid loss and subsequent dehydration can occur among clients who have pneumonia due to tachypnea, fever, and anorexia.

2. Fluid loss and subsequent dehydration can occur among clients who have meningitis due to fever and vomiting.

4. Clients who have elevated blood glucose may become dehydrated. Fluid will be lost via the kidneys as excess glucose is excreted.

Nursing Process: Analyzing
Client Need: Physiological Integrity

8 - 4 2

③ **When monitoring the irrigation, the nurse should check to be sure that the solution out-flow corresponds to the irrigation inflow and patency of the catheter is maintained. Continuous bladder irrigations require a steady flow of fluids into the bladder. Fluid entering the bladder and fluid draining from the bladder should be in appropriate proportions (equal amounts).**

1. The bladder irrigation should be continuous.
2. The irrigations should be continuous and should flow by gravity.
4. The irrigating solution should be administered at room temperature.

Nursing Process: Implementing
Client Need: Physiological Integrity

8 - 4 3

③ **Peritoneal dialysis utilizes the peritoneum as a semipermeable membrane. The dialysate dwells in the abdominal cavity and exchange takes place through the peritoneum.**

1. The dialysate dwells in the abdominal cavity that surrounds the intestines; it does not dwell in the intestines.
2. Peritoneal dialysis may be used indefinitely if it is successful and remains free of infection.
4. The complete peritoneal dialysis takes several times longer than hemodialysis and often requires several changes.

Nursing Process: Implementing
Client Need: Physiological Integrity

8 - 4 4

② **When administering sodium polystyrene sulfonate, the nurse will expect the desired therapeutic effect to occur through decreased potassium intoxication. Sodium polystyrene sulfonate (Kayexalate) is an ion-exchange resin that removes potassium (K+) from the gastrointestinal tract. The resins, which are not absorbed in the gastrointestinal tract, exchange sodium (Na+) and hydrogen (H+) for potassium (K+). Potassium is then excreted in the feces.**

1. The desired therapeutic effect of sodium polystyrene sulfonate will not occur via shifts in intracellular potassium because the ion exchange is effective only in the gastrointestinal tract.

3 and 4. Sodium polystyrene sulfonate (kayexalate) has no impact on serum level of sodium or sulfate.

Nursing Process: Implementing
Client Need: Physiological Integrity

8 - 4 5

④ **The signs of fluid overload are coughing and wheezing. A cough and wheeze may be due to the buildup of fluid in the lungs that can occur if excess intravenous fluids are administered. Other signs and symptoms of fluid overload include headache, hyponatremia, distended neck veins, and rapid breathing.**

1. Weight gain (not loss) would indicate fluid overload.

2. An increase (not decrease) in blood pressure would indicate fluid overload.

3. An increase (not decrease) in respiratory rate would indicate fluid overload. An increase in the respiratory rate would increase insensible loss of fluid and would be considered a compensatory mechanism in response to fluid overload.

Nursing Process: Analyzing

Client Need: Physiological Integrity

8 - 4 6

② **The nurse should question a 2000-calorie, high-carbohydrate, high-protein diet. Dietary protein is usually limited in acute renal failure to decrease nitrogenous metabolic waste products.**

1. Polystyrene sodium sulfonate (Kayexalate) reduces serum potassium by exchanging sodium for potassium ions in the gastrointestinal tract. Because the client is hyperkalemic and hyponatremic, this is a reasonable prescription. Normal potassium is 3.5 to 55 mEq/liter. Normal sodium is 135 to 145 mEq/liter.

3. Hypertonic glucose and Regular insulin promote movement of potassium into the cells. This will reduce hyperkalemia.

4. Fluid imbalance must be carefully monitored. Intake should be only slightly more than output per 24 hours. Intake is frequently based on prior 8-hour output.

Nursing Process: Evaluating

Client Need: Safe, Effective Care Environment

8 - 4 7

③ **A low urine volume will increase the risk of nephrolithiasis. Nephrolithiasis (kidney stones) are formed from the salts of urine. The incidence is related to sex, race, diet, and geographic location.**

1. Men are more prone to develop kidney stones than women.

2. Persons of European descent tend to have a higher incidence than persons of African descent.

4. Kidney stones are not associated with pain until they become lodged in a portion of the urinary tract.

Nursing Process: Evaluating

Client Need: Physiological Integrity

8 - 4 8

②　**Although the catheter appears to be draining well, gentle palpation can be used to further assess the client for bladder fullness.**

1.　Pinkish-red urine with small clots is a normal finding at this time.

3.　The catheter is usually positioned to pull the retention balloon into the prostatic fossa to provide hemostasis following a transurethral resection of the prostate.

4.　Attempting to void around the catheter causes the bladder muscles to contract and produces painful "bladder spasms." The client should be instructed not to bear down in an attempt to void around the catheter.

Nursing Process:　Implementing

Client Need:　Health Promotion and Maintenance

Practice Test 9

Reproductive System

9 - 1

Should your pregnant client have an increase in femoral venous pressure, your assessment would most likely reveal:

1. varicose veins.
2. urinary frequency.
3. pain in the calf of the leg upon dorsal flexion of the foot when the leg is extended.
4. relatively painless contractions of the uterus that are not associated with labor.

9 - 2

Your client has just experienced a radical mastectomy. Which instruction should be given to the client to help avoid complications associated with lymphedema?

1. Wear a tight elastic wrap on your arm during the day.
2. Keep your arm as immobile as possible.
3. Avoid any exposure to sunlight on your arm.
4. Gradually increase your arm's exercise, but avoid heavy lifting.

9 - 3

Your client says she felt a gush of fluid from her vagina. After determining that the client's membranes have ruptured, your first action would be to:

1. clean the client and provide a dry gown.
2. assist the client to the bathroom and help her clean up.
3. assess fetal heart tones.
4. assess maternal vital signs.

9 - 4

A 41-week gravida III comes to the labor and delivery unit crying and holding her abdomen. She has been having contractions for 8 hours at home with pain in her lower back. On palpation, her contractions are very intense and 5 minutes apart, but she is only dilated 2 cm. The physician prescribed oxytocin intravenous to:

1. increase duration of contractions.
2. increase resting tone.
3. decrease intensity of contractions.
4. increase uterine activity.

9 - 5

You are preparing a client in her twenty-third week of gestation for an amniocentesis during her next scheduled clinic appointment. You inform the client that on the day of the amniocentesis, she should:

1. refrain from eating.
2. take an enema.
3. empty the bladder.
4. cleanse the abdomen.

9 - 6

A client reaches 4 cm dilatation and asks for an epidural. Following administration of an epidural, the nurse will assess the client for the common side effect of:

1. hypotension.
2. hypertension.
3. headache.
4. dyspnea.

9 - 7

Upon reviewing the laboratory results of a client in her thirty-second week of pregnancy, you observe the hemoglobin to be 11.6 g/dL. Her pre-pregnancy hemoglobin is 13.6 g/dL. You know the decrease in the client's hemoglobin is because:

1. the placenta destroys many maternal blood cells.
2. insidious blood loss is occurring.
3. the stress of pregnancy has probably caused a gastric ulcer to form.
4. the pregnant woman's plasma volume has increased, but the number of her red blood cells is probably the same.

9 - 8

The most typical sign of primary syphilis is:

1. painful, clustered vesicles on the genitalia.
2. rash and flulike symptoms.
3. cardiovascular involvement.
4. painless chancre on the genitalia.

9 - 9

Your client's contractions are 5 to 7 minutes apart, she is dilated 2 cm, and the baby is at the -1 station. This means the presenting part is:

1. 1 cm below the ischial spine.
2. in the pelvic outlet.
3. at the level of the ischial spine.
4. moving into mid pelvis.

9 - 1 0

Women who have had total hysterectomies, including removal of both ovaries, should be encouraged to take:

1. estrogen.
2. calcium.
3. progesterone.
4. vitamin B12 by injection.

9 - 1 1

A pregnant client has chlamydia. The nurse will teach the client that:

1. chlamydia is not a sexually transmitted disease.
2. persons with chlamydia are carriers of the disease throughout their lives.
3. chlamydia is treated with antiviral medications.
4. the treatment of choice for chlamydia is erythromycin 250 mg po q 6 hours.

9 - 1 2

A client had a vasectomy at a local clinic. You are reviewing postoperative home care instructions with the client and his wife. Which of the following comments by the client's wife would indicate the need for review of basic information regarding a postoperative vasectomy?

1. "I'm glad I didn't throw out your old athletic support."
2. "Having so much football on TV this week should help. He can rest on the couch and watch TV."
3. "It's lucky that golf tournament he wanted to play in is 2 weeks away. Maybe he won't have to miss it."
4. "Talk about nice timing. I just finished my last pack of birth control pills."

9 - 1 3

A client in her thirty-sixth week of gestation has premature rupture of the amniotic membranes. The nurse will give priority to which goal?

1. helping the client remain free of infection
2. reaching the client's lecithin/sphin-gomyelin (L/S) ratio of 2:1
3. helping the client demonstrate effective coping abilities
4. helping the client remain free of discomfort

9 - 1 4

A client's Papanicolaou smear indicated the presence of dysplasia. You explain to the client that this indicates:

1. a decrease in the size or number of cells.
2. an increase in the size of cells.
3. an increase in the number of cells.
4. a change in the size, shape, and appearance of the cells.

9 - 1 5

A client had a dilatation and curettage under general anesthesia. The results of blood work drawn during surgery include a red blood count of 2,500,000 per cu/mm of blood. Which action should the nurse take?

1. Notify the nurse in charge about laboratory results.
2. Force fluids to 2000 cc per 24 hours.
3. Encourage the client to rest as much as possible.
4. Continue with the client's established plan of care.

9 - 1 6

Screening tests for cancer such as the Papanicolaou test or mammogram are considered to be which form of intervention?

1. acute
2. primary
3. secondary
4. tertiary

9 - 1 7

A 46-year-old male who has just had a routine pre-employment physical had the following laboratory results. Which laboratory finding warrants further and prompt investigation?

1. hemoglobin (hgb) 14.8 g/dL
2. white blood count 7500/cm³
3. prostate specific antigen 19.6 ng/ml
4. bilirubin 0.6 mg/dL

9 - 1 8

Which of the following doses of ethinyl estradiol would be most appropriate to start with for an 18-year-old female experiencing dysmenorrhea?

1. 5 µg
2. 35 µg
3. 65 µg
4. 5 µg

9 - 1 9

A postmenopausal client with no surgical history inquires about the benefits of taking daily estrogen versus an estrogen and progesterone combination. You know the reason for the combination is:

1. fertility is maintained with the combination.
2. estrogen alone will cause hirsutism and acne.
3. regular menstrual cycles resume with combination therapy.
4. progesterone will prevent hyperproliferation of the uterus.

9 - 2 0

The exogenous administration of glucocorticoids is usually done:

1. to promote diuresis.
2. for their anti-inflammatory effects.
3. for their analgesic properties.
4. for their antiarrhythmic properties.

9-21

Which of the following is the most common cause of secondary amenorrhea?

1. gonadal dysgenesis
2. imperforate hymen
3. anorexia nervosa
4. pregnancy

9-22

The nurse has been teaching a prenatal client pelvic-tilt exercises. This intervention can be considered effective if the client experiences a decrease in:

1. leg cramps.
2. backaches.
3. hemorrhoids.
4. constipation.

9-23

You are teaching the mother of a term newborn how to care for her infant. Which statement made by the mother indicates a need for further teaching?

1. "My baby may have dark, tarry-looking stools for a few days."
2. "My baby may have some peeling of the hands and feet."
3. "Diaper rash may be prevented by using protective ointments."
4. "I should hold and talk to my baby during feeding."

9-24

Which hormone is responsible for the ejection of breast milk?

1. oxytocin
2. follicle-stimulating hormone
3. glucagon
4. thyrotropin

9 - 2 5

Which of the following conditions would most likely be the cause of infertility in the male?

1. pertussis
2. mumps
3. varicella
4. pneumonia

9 - 2 6

Which manifestation is not an indication for a hysterectomy?

1. uterine prolapse repair
2. dysfunctional uterine bleeding
3. sterilization
4. uterine cancer

9 - 2 7

Postmenopausal hormone replacement therapy has which of the following effects on both high-density lipoprotein (HDL) and low-density lipoprotein (LDL)?

1. Hormone replacement therapy increases HDL and decreases LDL.
2. Hormone replacement therapy increases HDL and increases LDL.
3. Hormone replacement therapy decreases HDL and decreases LDL.
4. Hormone replacement therapy decreases HDL and increases LDL.

9 - 2 8

Which finding would interfere the most with the continuation of a pregnancy?

1. an increase in human chorionic gonadotropin
2. an increase in follicle-stimulating hormone
3. a decrease in alpha-fetoprotein
4. a decrease in progesterone

9 - 2 9

Teaching a client arm-strengthening exercises during the postmastectomy period is considered which of the following forms of intervention?

1. acute
2. primary
3. secondary
4. tertiary

9 - 3 0

A client at 12 weeks' gestation has hyperemesis gravidarum. Which assessment will provide the most relevant information about the client's condition?

1. intake and output
2. fetal heart rate
3. activity level
4. emotional state

9 - 3 1

A client with genital herpes has been instructed concerning methods that will prevent transmission of that condition. Upon entering the client's room, the nurse observes the client's friend coming out of the bathroom. Which action would be essential for the nurse to take first?

1. Report the incident to the nurse in charge.
2. Record the incident in the nurses' notes.
3. Reinforce precaution instructions to the client and the client's friend.
4. Discuss precaution instructions with the client after the friend leaves.

9 - 3 2

A client is scheduled for a dilatation and curettage. Preoperative prescriptions include secobarbital po at bedtime. In addition to promoting sleep, the nurse understands that secobarbital is given to:

1. reduce the client's anxiety level.
2. lessen bronchial secretions.
3. decrease the muscle tone of the uterus.
4. minimize the need for postoperative analgesia.

9 - 3 3

A client with placenta previa had a cesarean section performed under spinal block anesthesia. A 4-pound (1814 g) infant was delivered and placed in an incubator in the premature nursery. Which action should be given priority when planning the client's postoperative care?

1. Instruct the client to lie flat in the bed for at least 6 hours.
2. Allow the client to see the infant as soon as possible.
3. Record the client's intake and output.
4. Assess for muscle fatigue.

9 - 3 4

The contraceptive levonorgestrel should be used cautiously by a client who:

1. has just completed a round of tetracycline.
2. is 26 years of age.
3. takes phenytoin.
4. smokes cigarettes.

9 - 3 5

The nurse is caring for a client in a post-partum clinic. Which manifestations would indicate the presence of an abnormality?

1. a chill shortly after delivery
2. a pulse rate of 60 the morning after delivery
3. urinary output of 3000 ml the second day after delivery
4. oral temperature of 101°F the third day after delivery

9 - 3 6

Your client was hospitalized with a suspected incomplete abortion. She has abdominal pain and a moderate amount of vaginal bleeding. Which action would be most important to include in the client's nursing-care plan?

1. restriction of food and fluids
2. observation of amount and type of vaginal bleeding
3. instructions on birth control methods
4. limitation of activity until pain and bleeding cease

9 - 3 7

A client with a third-degree episiotomy and hemorrhoids is concerned that she might become constipated. You will advise the client to:

1. eat fruit with each meal.
2. increase intake of drinks with caffeine.
3. decrease intake of high-protein foods.
4. increase dairy product intake.

9 - 3 8

A 56-year-old client is on a low-dose estrogen therapy to manage osteoporosis. Which of the following statements reflects the nurse's knowledge of the complications of estrogen replacement therapy?

1. She needs to use contraceptives to avoid pregnancy.
2. She needs to call her physician if she experiences any breathing difficulties.
3. It is important to have regular gynecological checkups.
4. She may need to consider plastic surgery for varicosities common with estrogen therapy.

9 - 3 9

A client in her twelfth week of gestation calls the physician's office and tells the nurse that she just had an episode of bleeding. The nurse determines that the client had a moderate amount of reddish-brown mucous discharge. Which action should the nurse take first?

1. Determine if the client has transportation and recommend that she see the physician.
2. Assure the client she has nothing to worry about and suggest she call if the bleeding gets worse.
3. Ask the client to lie down for an hour and then call to report what happens with the bleeding.
4. Tell the client that it sounds as though she has been too active and suggest she rest more throughout her pregnancy.

9 - 4 0

A mother is bottle-feeding her baby. On the third day postpartum, she develops engorgement in both breasts. The nurse should advise the mother to:

1. apply warm compresses to her breasts.
2. use an electric breast pump to empty her breasts.
3. apply a tight binder and apply ice packs to her breasts.
4. manually express the milk while taking a warm shower.

9 - 4 1

A 24-year-old gravida I with a history of mitral valve prolapse presents for delivery. Because of the rapid fluid shift that takes place following the delivery, the nurse would carefully observe for symptoms of:

1. endocarditis.
2. pulmonary embolism.
3. congestive heart failure.
4. pregnancy-induced hypertension.

9 - 4 2

A client with severe preeclampsia has been placed on the external fetal monitor. Moderate uterine contractions are occurring every 5 minutes, 50 to 60 seconds in duration. In view of the client's preeclampsia, which of the following should the nurse recognize as an ominous sign that must be monitored closely?

1. severe epigastric pain
2. urinary output of 60 cc per hour
3. 1+ protein in the urine
4. facial edema

9 - 4 3

A mother had a cesarean section and was transferred to the postpartum unit from the recovery room. Postpartum nursing management of this client includes administration of bromocriptine mesylate. The nurse should expect that this medication was prescribed to:

1. promote sodium retention.
2. suppress the production of chorionic gonadotropin.
3. inhibit secretion of the lactogenic hormone.
4. diminish lochial flow.

9 - 4 4

A client in her eighth month of pregnancy has been hospitalized with preeclampsia. One morning she tells the nurse she thinks her contractions are beginning. Which of the following approaches should the nurse use to fully assess the presence of uterine contractions?

1. Place the hands on opposite sides of the upper part of the abdomen and curve them somewhat around the uterine fundus.
2. Place the heel of the hand on the abdomen just above the umbilicus and press firmly.
3. Place the hand flat on the abdomen over the uterine fundus, with the fingers apart, pressing slightly.
4. Place the hand in the middle of the upper abdomen and then move the hand several times to different parts of the abdomen.

9 - 4 5

Your client has missed 1 menstrual period and comes to the physician's office for a pregnancy test. The client's pregnancy test is positive. You recognize this is a:

1. presumptive sign.
2. probable sign.
3. diagnostic sign.
4. subjective sign.

9 - 4 6

A 16-year-old high school student attends the antepartal clinic on a regular basis. She is a gravida I at 28 weeks' gestation. The nurse assesses her to determine if she is retaining abnormal amounts of fluid. Which of the following findings would be indicative of a nursing diagnosis of "alteration in fluid volume, excess"?

1. She has gained 3 lbs (1361 g) during the past week.
2. She has gained 4.5 lbs (2041 g) over the past month.
3. She has gained 11 lbs (4990 g) in the second trimester of pregnancy.
4. She has gained 14 lbs (6350 g) since the onset of pregnancy.

9 - 4 7

A primigravida in her thirty-sixth week of gestation comes to the Emergency Department. The client is experiencing profuse painless vaginal bleeding. The primary nursing diagnosis at this time would be:

1. fear related to personal safety and safety of the fetus.
2. potential preterm delivery related to vaginal bleeding.
3. potential for infection related to loss of mucus plug.
4. altered tissue perfusion secondary to excessive blood loss.

9 - 4 8

Your client is 4 hours post cesarean section. Her vital signs are stable and she is receiving intravenous therapy. Interventions for the nursing diagnosis, altered perfusion related to excessive blood loss, would include:

1. turn, cough, and deep breathe every 2 hours.
2. evaluate firmness and position of fundus.
3. administer analgesic medications.
4. massage uterus every 30 minutes.

9 - 4 9

Which of the following responses by the nurse reflects an understanding of couvade, Mitleiden, or "suffering along" often experienced by expectant fathers?

1. "The symptoms that are felt will increase throughout the wife's pregnancy."
2. "Some men actually believe they are pregnant."
3. "Many expectant fathers have physical symptoms associated with their partner's pregnancy."
4. "You are getting an example of what happens to a pregnant woman."

9 - 5 0

The most common side effect to assess following the administration of an epidural is:

1. hypotension.
2. hypertension.
3. headache.
4. dyspnea.

Practice Test 9

Answers, Rationales, and Explanations

9 - 1

(1) **Your assessment would most likely reveal varicose veins. Clients who are pregnant may have an increase in femoral venous pressure. An increase in femoral pressure will distend the veins and could cause varicose veins. Increased circulating volume and hormonal relaxation of the blood vessel walls contribute to vascular wall distention and elevated venous stasis or varicosities.**

2. An increase in femoral venous pressure does not put pressure on the bladder.

3. Pain in the calf of the leg upon dorsal flexion of the foot when the leg is extended (Homans' sign) is a sign of deep vein thrombosis.

4. Braxton-Hicks contractions are painless and irregular. They occur throughout pregnancy and may enhance placental blood flow.

Nursing Process: Assessing

Client Need: Health Promotion and Maintenance

9 - 2

(4) **Clients experiencing a radical mastectomy should gradually increase arm exercises and avoid heavy lifting. Clients experiencing a radical mastectomy have not only had breast tissue and muscle removed, but have more than likely had lymph nodes and some lymph channels removed. In order to promote the circulation of lymph in this compromised lymph system, moderate range-of-motion exercise should be encouraged. Actions that compromise circulation, such as heavy lifting or tight gripping, should be avoided.**

1 and 2. Compression and immobility tend to decrease, not increase, circulation to the affected area and would therefore be contraindicated.

3. There is no positive correlation between moderate exposure to light and compromise of lymph circulation.

Nursing Process: Implementing

Client Need: Physiological Integrity

9 - 3

(3) **The nurse will assess the fetal heart tones to ensure that the umbilical cord has not prolapsed and compromised the fetus.**

1. The client can be cleaned up after determining fetal well-being.

2. Once the amniotic sac has ruptured, the mother should remain in bed to prevent the possibility of a prolapsed umbilical cord.

4. The maternal vital signs would be assessed after the fetal heart tones have been evaluated. Once the amniotic sac ruptures, it is the fetus, not the mother, who could be compromised.

Nursing Process: Implementing

Client Need: Health Promotion and Maintenance

9 - 4

④ **The physician prescribed oxytocin (Pitocin) intravenously to increase uterine activity and promote more effective contractions. The client is experiencing dystocia (ineffective uterine contractions) caused by dysfunctional labor.**

1. The problem is not duration of the client's contractions but the fact that the contractions are ineffective.

2. The frequency of the client's contractions is 5 minutes. This suggests that there is enough resting tone between contractions for the uterus to relax and the placenta to be profused. What is needed is increased uterine activity.

3. Oxytocin was prescribed to increase uterine activity, not decrease intensity of contractions.

Nursing Process: Analyzing

Client Need: Physiological Integrity

9 - 5

③ **You will instruct the client to empty her bladder prior to the amniocentesis. Since the bladder lies in the anterior pelvic cavity, it should be emptied prior to the amniocentesis to prevent possible puncture or displacement of the uterine cavity and fetus. An amniocentesis involves inserting a needle through the maternal abdomen into the uterine cavity to collect a sample of amniotic fluid.**

1. It is not necessary to be npo for an amniocentesis. The procedure is performed using a local anesthetic.

2. It is not necessary to have an enema. The gastrointestinal tract is not involved.

4. The client will not need to cleanse her abdomen. The nurse will prep the abdomen with a cleansing agent immediately before the procedure.

Nursing Process: Implementing

Client Need: Safe, Effective Care Environment

9 - 6

① **Following the administration of an epidural, the most common side effect is hypotension due to diminished vasomotor tone. During the postblock phase, the nurse will closely monitor the mother's cardiovascular and ventilatory integrity.**

2. Hypotension, not hypertension, is the most common side effect.

3. Headaches will not occur because the epidural is in the dural space.

4. Some difficulty in breathing could occur but this is not a common side effect.

Nursing Process: Assessing

Client Need: Physiological Integrity

9 - 7

④ **A normal occurrence during pregnancy is an increase in plasma volume. As a result, a physiologic anemia occurs. A physiologic anemia is due to an increase in plasma volume, not a decrease in the actual red blood cells. The opposite may be true of a dehydrated person, who may have an elevated hemoglobin due to hemoconcentration.**

1. The placenta does not destroy maternal red blood cells.
2. Blood loss is both uncommon and untoward during pregnancy.
3. Gastric ulcers are not known to be formed due to the stress of pregnancy, although heartburn and reflux are common complaints.

Nursing Process: Evaluating
Client Need: Health Promotion and Maintenance

9 - 8

④ **The most typical sign of primary syphilis is a painless chancre on the genitalia. Syphilis is characterized by three distinct stages. Primary syphilis usually presents itself with a painless chancre on the genitalia that may go unnoticed. Secondary syphilis is often flu-like in nature, involving generalized fatigue, rash, and fever. Latent syphilis, which may not present itself for years, involves the whole body and may present itself with confusion, muscle weakness, and cardiovascular involvement.**

1. Primary syphilis usually presents itself with a painless chancre on the genitalia.
2. The rash and flulike symptoms are more common to secondary syphilis.
3. The neurological and cardiovascular involvement of this disease is usually seen during the latent phase.

Nursing Process: Evaluating
Client Need: Physiological Integrity

9 - 9

④ **When the presenting part is at the –1 station, the fetus is said to be moving from the pelvic inlet to the mid pelvis.**

1. The level of the ischial spine would be zero station.
2. If the fetus were in the pelvic outlet, the station would be positive.
3. Since the fetus is at the -1 station, it is actually 1 cm above the ischial spine.

Nursing Process: Assessing
Client Need: Physiological Integrity

9 - 1 0

① Women who have had total hysterectomies, including removal of both ovaries, should be encouraged to take estrogen. Estrogen is produced and secreted by the ovaries. This hormone is not only responsible for maintaining portions of the menstrual cycle but is also associated with bone density and a decrease in cardiac risk factors for premenstrual women. Women who have lost their ovarian function are most often encouraged to continue endogenous hormone replacement.

2 and 4. Calcium and vitamin B12 levels are not directly associated with ovarian function.

3. Progesterone is important in preventing hyperproliferation of the uterus and in the onset of menses. In the absence of a uterus, this role wouldn't be applicable.

Nursing Process: Planning

Client Need: Health Promotion and Maintenance

9 - 1 1

④ The treatment of choice for pregnant women with chlamydia is erythromycin (Erythrozone) 250 mg po q 6 hours for 7 days. Chlamydia is a sexually transmitted disease caused by the bacterium *Chlamydia trachomatis*. It is highly contagious.

1. The nurse should teach the client that chlamydia is a sexually transmitted disease.

2. Chlamydia can be treated successfully. People who have chlamydia and are treated effectively are not carriers of the disease.

3. Chlamydia is not caused by a virus. It is caused by the bacterium *Chlamydia trachomatis* and is treated by anti-infectives.

Nursing Process: Implementing

Client Need: Physiological Integrity

9 - 1 2

④ The client's wife needs a basic review regarding a postoperative vasectomy. Sperm remain in the semen beyond the point of occlusion of the vas deferens and only gradually disappear from the ejaculate. An alternate method of contraception should be used until semen analysis confirms absence of sperm from the ejaculate. It usually takes 15 to 20 ejaculations or 4 to 6 weeks before all sperm are removed form the proximal portions of the sperm ducts.

1. A support for the scrotum is helpful following a vasectomy. Ice packs may also be applied to reduce swelling and relieve discomfort.

2. It is recommended that the client rest a few days following a vasectomy. Lying on the sofa would probably be beneficial.

3. The client should be able to participate in a golf tournament 2 weeks post surgically without any problem.

Nursing Process: Evaluating

Client Need: Health Promotion and Maintenance

9 - 1 3

   ① Keeping the client free from infection is essential since bacteria may travel upward into the uterus and compromise the well-being of the fetus. Because of the break in the surface of the amniotic membranes, the client will be at risk for infection.

2. At 35 weeks of gestation, the lecithin/sphingomyelin (L/S) ratio should have already reached 2:1. Therefore, the L/S ratio will not be a consideration.

3. It is important for the client to cope effectively. However, keeping the mother and fetus free from infection is the primary goal.

4. Premature rupture of the amniotic membranes does not produce pain.

Nursing Process: Planning
Client Need: Safe, Effective Care Environment

9 - 1 4

   ④ You explain that dysplasia is bizarre cell growth that results in cells that differ in size, shape, and appearance from other cells of the same tissue.

1. Atrophy is a decrease in the size or number of cells that primarily affects skeletal muscle and secondary sex organs.

2. Hypertrophy is an increase in the size of cells and hence the size of the organs they form.

3. Hyperplasia is an increase in the number of cells in an organ or tissue. As the cells multiply, volume increases.

Nursing Process: Evaluating
Client Need: Physiological Integrity

9 - 1 5

   ① The nurse should notify the nurse in charge. The normal range for red blood cells in a healthy adult female is 4,500,000 to 5,000,000 cu/mm. Since 2,500,000 is significantly lower than normal, this must be brought to the attention of the nurse in charge so further instructions for care may be obtained.

2. Forcing fluids may increase the client's circulating fluid volume but the client needs the oxygen-carrying capacity of the red blood cells. Also, increasing fluids under the circumstances could cause nausea, vomiting, and possible aspiration.

3. Rest alone will not increase the number of red blood cells needed to prevent the development of hemorrhagic shock.

4. The plan of care should be modified to meet the client's immediate needs.

Nursing Process: Implementing
Client Need: Physiological Integrity

9 - 1 6

③ **Secondary interventions are those that diagnose and treat illness. Because screening tests, such as the Papanicolanaou (PAP) test, are done specifically to diagnose an illness and have no real action in preventing the illness from occurring, they are considered to be secondary interventions.**

1. Acute interventions are those that act immediately on a disease process and are considered in the realm of secondary interventions.

2. Primary interventions such as immunizations or wellness teaching prevent disease.

4. Tertiary interventions, such as cardiac rehabilitation, are those that help in the recovery process of an illness or injury.

Nursing Process: Assessing
Client Need: Physiological Integrity

9 - 1 7

③ **Prostate specific antigen of 19.6 ng/ml would warrant prompt investigation. Prostate specific antigen (PSA) is a protease secreted by the prostate gland only. Serum PSA levels above 10 ng/ml are considered abnormally elevated. Elevations may be due to conditions such as benign prostatic hypertrophy or may be due to a tumor in the prostate.**

1, 2, and 4. A hemoglobin of 14.8 g/dL is within the normal range for men (range is 14 to 18 g/dL), a white blood cell count of 7,500/cm^3 is within the normal range (range is 5000 to 10,000 cm^3), and a bilirubin of 0.6 mg/dL is within the normal range (range is 0.1 to 1.0 mg/dL).

Nursing Process: Analyzing
Client Need: Physiological Integrity

9 - 1 8

② **Ethinyl estradiol is a synthetic estrogen and a major component of most oral contraceptives presently on the market. The common dosage of the pill is usually 35 μg to 50 μg. Usually, a young client is started on the smaller dose, then the dose is increased as necessary.**

1, 3, and 4. There is no commonly marketed birth control pill containing 5 μg or 65 μg of ethinyl estradiol and 5 mg represents 5,000 μg, a grossly excessive dosage.

Nursing Process: Implementing
Client Need: Safe, Effective Care Environment

9 - 1 9

④ **Progesterone will prevent hyperproliferation of the uterus. Estrogen hormone replacement therapy alone may cause hyperproliferation of the uterus, which markedly increases the risk of uterine cancer. As a general rule, only women without uteruses may take estrogen alone as their postmenopausal hormone replacement.**

1, 2, and 3. The intent of postmenopausal hormone replacement is not fertility, but cardioprotective and orthopedic benefits. Estrogen therapy is not related to hirsutism and acne (the androgen hormones are) and regular menstrual cycles do not resume with the combination therapy (that is more likely to occur with estrogen alone).

Nursing Process: Analyzing
Client Need: Physiological Integrity

9 - 2 0

② **The exogenous administration of glucocorticoids is usually done for their anti-inflammatory effects. Systemic administration of glucocorticoids may be used in allergic reactions or inflammatory disorders. Glucocorticoids such as cortisol are produced by the adrenal cortex and affect metabolism and inflammation.**

1, 3, and 4. The glucocorticoids have neither diuretic, analgesic, or antiarrhythmic properties.

Nursing Process: Implementing
Client Need: Physiological Integrity

9 - 2 1

④ **The most common cause of secondary amenorrhea is pregnancy. Secondary amenorrhea is the absence of menses after menstrual cycles have been established. Other causes may include infection, hormonal disturbance, and starvation.**

1, 2, and 3. Turner's syndrome (gonadal dysgenesis) and imperforate hymen cause primary amenorrhea (no history of menses). Anorexia nervosa is a cause of secondary amenorrhea, but is not as common as pregnancy.

Nursing Process: Assessing
Client Need: Physiological Integrity

9-22

② **Pelvic-tilt exercises can be beneficial in preventing or relieving backaches in pregnant women. In nonpregnant women, pelvic tilting is useful in relieving menstrual cramps.**

1. Leg cramps may be prevented or relieved by dorsiflexion and plantar flexion of the foot in combination with ankle rotation.

3 and 4. To prevent or minimize hemorrhoids, one should avoid constipation by maintaining regular bowel habits, drinking plenty of fluids, and providing fiber in the diet.

Nursing Process: Implementing
Client Need: Physiological Integrity

9-23

① **A newborn should not have dark, tarry-looking stools for several days. Meconium stools usually last from 12 to 24 hours. The first meconium passed is sterile but within hours all meconium contains bacteria. The first passage occurs within 24 hours in 90% of normal infants.**

2. Some peeling of the hands and feet is common in term newborns. However, thick, cracking, parchment-like skin is characteristic of the postterm newborn. The skin of the preterm newborn is smooth and thin enough to visualize blood vessels.

3. Diaper rash may be prevented by using protective ointment.

4. The infant should be held and "talked to" when feeding. This will promote socialization.

Nursing Process: Implementing
Client Need: Health Promotion and Maintenance

9-24

① **The hormone responsible for the ejection of breast milk is oxytocin. Oxytocin is secreted by the pituitary gland and is responsible for the ejection of breast milk and contractions of the uterus. Prolactin, also secreted by the pituitary gland, plays a role in milk secretion.**

2. Follicle-stimulating hormone (FSH) is responsible for the secretion of estrogen.

3. Glucagon increases blood sugar.

4. Thyrotropin stimulates the thyroid gland.

Nursing Process: Evaluating
Client Need: Health Promotion and Maintenance

9 - 2 5

② The most likely cause of infertility in the male is mumps. Men who contract mumps during adulthood have a higher incidence of sterility. Mumps is a viral infection that typically affects the salivary glands—hence the classic swollen jaws associated with this disease. Its complications include central nervous system involvement, kidney infections, pancreas infection, and infection of the testicles.

1, 3, and 4. Neither pertussis (whooping cough), varicella (chicken pox), or pneumonia are directly associated with male sterility.

Nursing Process: Evaluating
Client Need: Physiological Integrity

9 - 2 6

③ Sterilization may be accomplished by hysterectomy, but it is not an indication for hysterectomy in the absence of pathology. The most appropriate surgical sterilization procedure for the female client is tubal ligation. Tubal ligation is a less extensive surgery and has a lower morbidity and mortality rate.

1, 2, and 4. The removal of the uterus may be indicated in the instance of extreme uterine prolapse; dysfunctional uterine bleeding that doesn't respond to pharmacological measures; and uterine cancer.

Nursing Process: Assessing
Client Need: Physiological Integrity

9 - 2 7

① Estrogen replacement affects how the body metabolizes fats. High-density lipoproteins increase and low-density lipoproteins decrease. The overall effect is that the risk of heart disease is decreased in postmenopausal women who are on hormone replacement.

2, 3, and 4. Hormone replacement therapy tends to increase HDL levels and decrease LDL levels.

Nursing Process: Evaluating
Client Need: Health Promotion and Maintenance

9-28

④ **A decrease in progesterone would interfere the most with the continuation of pregnancy. Progesterone is needed to maintain a pregnancy.**

1. Human chorionic gonadotrophin (HGG) is a hormone of pregnancy and will increase.

2. Follicle-stimulating hormone (FHS) will increase.

3. A decrease in alpha-fetoprotein (AFP) may indicate a problem such as Down syndrome. A decrease in AFP is seen in high-risk pregnancy.

Nursing Process: Planning

Client Need: Safe, Effective Care Environment

9-29

④ **Tertiary interventions, such as rehabilitation from a mastectomy, heart attack, or diabetes diagnoses, are those that help in the recovery process of an illness or injury.**

1, 2, and 3. Acute and secondary interventions, such as medication administration and screening, are those used in the diagnosis and treatment of an illness. Primary interventions , such as immunizations, are those that are used in the prevention of illness.

Nursing Process: Planning

Client Need: Health Promotion and Maintenance

9-30

① **Intake and output will provide the most relevant information about the status of a client with hyperemesis gravidarum. Hyperemesis gravidarum is characterized by intractable vomiting during pregnancy. It results in dehydration and electrolyte imbalance.**

2. The fetal heart rate would provide information about the status of the fetus but would not provide any information about the status of women with hyperemesis gravidarum.

3 and 4. The activity level and emotional state of the client would provide some information about how the client is feeling generally, but it would not indicate the status of the client with hyperemesis gravidarum.

Nursing Process: Assessing

Client Need: Health Promotion and Maintenance

9 - 3 1

③ **The best way to handle the problem is to discuss the problem with the client and the client's friend. Toilet isolation is one method used to prevent the spread of genital herpes.**

1 and 2. Reporting the incident to the nurse in charge and recording it in the client's chart can be done after reinforcing precautions that should be taken to prevent the spread or reinfection of the client and the client's friend.

4. The client's friend needs to be taught what precautions should be taken to prevent the spread of the disease.

Nursing Process: Implementing

Client Need: Safe, Effective Care Environment

9 - 3 2

① **Secobarbital is given to reduce the client's anxiety. Secobarbital (Seconal) is a short-acting barbiturate that works as a central nervous system depressant. It is administered to a client scheduled for surgery to produce mild sedation, thus reducing the level of the client's anxiety.**

2. Secobarbital (Seconal) is a short-acting barbiturate and does not affect bronchial secretions. Atropine, an anticholinergic, is a common medication administered shortly before surgery that decreases oral and respiratory secretions.

3. Secobarbital (Seconal) does not affect uterine muscle tone.

4. The effects of secobarbital (Seconal) will have worn off by the time the client has had the dilatation and curettage (D & C). The onset of po secobarbital (Seconal) is 15 minutes, peak effect 15 to 30 minutes, and duration 1 to 4 hours.

Nursing Process: Evaluating

Client Need: Physiological Integrity

9 - 3 3

① **The client should be instructed to lie flat in bed for at least 6 hours. Spinal anesthesia may cause a headache due to the potential for leakage of the cerebral spinal fluid through the needle tract in the dura. To prevent leakage, the client should remain flat in bed, preferably prone.**

2. The client should see her infant as soon as possible. However, this is not a priority at this time.

3. A record of the client's intake and output will be maintained, but this is not the priority at this time.

4. Assessing the client's muscle fatigue is important but it is not the priority at this time.

Nursing Process: Planning

Client Need: Physiological Integrity

9 - 3 4

④ **Clients who smoke cigarettes while taking oral contraceptives may increase their risk of serious side effects. Contraindications for use of hormonal contraceptives include a history of thromboembolic disorders, cardiovascular disease, cerebrovascular disease, liver tumors, or gallbladder disease. Contraceptives including levonorgestrol (Norplant) should be used cautiously by those over 35 or with a history of cigarette smoking. Also, the drug's effectiveness may be decreased by anti-infectives and weight changes.**

1. Tetracycline would no longer be in the bloodstream 3 weeks after the last dosage taken. Clients are advised to use a second method of birth control if they are taking a contraceptive concurrently with an anti-infective.

2. This client's age (26) would not place her at risk if she chooses to use an oral or implanted contraceptive.

3. Clients who take phenytoin (Dilantin) are advised to use a second method of birth control. Dilantin compromises the effects of oral and implanted contraceptives.

Nursing Process: Implementing
Client Need: Health Promotion and Maintenance

9 - 3 5

④ **An oral body temperature of 101°F (38.3°C) on the third postpartal day indicates the probability of puerperal infection (septicemia following childbirth).**

1. A chill shortly after delivery is not considered pathologic. It is associated with muscle exhaustion, a sudden release of pressure off nerves following the birth of the fetus, and a response to epinephrine, if it is has been administered.

2. A pulse rate of 60 beats per minute the morning after delivery is not abnormal. This slow pulse rate is thought to be due to the hypervolemia that occurs after birth.

3. A urinary output of up to 3000 ml per day is normal following the delivery of a baby. This occurs as a consequence of an increase in the glomerular filtration rate and a decrease in progesterone, which has an antidiuretic effect.

Nursing Process: Collecting Data
Client Need: Safe, Effective Care Environment

9 - 3 6

② The nurse should include in the client's care plan the amount and type of vaginal bleeding. Bleeding may continue and cause severe hemorrhage until all products of conception have been expelled. The number of pads used and the amount and type of drainage should be recorded.

1. There is no need to restrict food and fluids. The client needs nourishment and plenty of fluids.

3. There is no indication that the client is interested in learning about birth control methods.

4. Limiting the client's activity will be instituted. However, assessing the amount and type of drainage is most important since severe hemorrhage could occur.

Nursing Process: Evaluating
Client Need: Physiological Integrity

9 - 3 7

① The client will be advised to eat fruit with each meal. Fruit will facilitate a normal bowel movement because of its fluid and fiber content.

2. Drinks with caffeine would not help to soften the stool and may cause upset stomach, nervousness, irritability, headache, and diarrhea.

3. Whereas high-protein foods would help in healing the episiotomy, they do not soften stools.

4. Dairy products contribute to constipation.

Nursing Process: Implementing
Client Need: Physiological Integrity

9 - 3 8

③ Women on low-dose estrogen therapy need to have regular gynecological checkups because they are at risk for uterine cancer; however, studies are unclear and further long-term studies are needed.

1, 2, and 4. Low-dose therapy does not predispose a postmenopausal woman to pregnancy, respiratory difficulties, or varicosities.

Nursing Process: Analyzing
Client Need: Health Promotion and Maintenance

9 - 3 9

③ **Many times, bleeding subsides with rest. The client needs to lie down for an hour and then call to report what is happening with the bleeding.**

1. Visiting the physician is unnecessary at this time.

2. Assuring the client there is "nothing to worry about" is belittling and blocks communication.

4. There is not enough evidence to support the need for bed rest throughout the pregnancy.

Nursing Process: Analyzing
Client Need: Physiological Integrity

9 - 4 0

③ **The client should be advised to apply a tight binder and apply ice packs to the breasts. Management of breast engorgement in the bottle-feeding mother is directed toward comfort measures that do not stimulate further milk production.**

1. Applying warm compresses to the mother's breasts will stimulate further milk production.

2. Using an electric pump to empty her breasts would stimulate further milk production.

4. Manually expressing milk from the mother's breasts while taking a warm shower will stimulate milk production.

Nursing Process: Implementing
Client Need: Health Promotion and Maintenance

9 - 4 1

③ **This 24-year-old gravida I with a history of mitral valve prolapse needs to be observed for congestive heart failure. The rapid shift of fluids following delivery places a great workload on the heart.**

1. Endocarditis refers to the lining membrane of the heart. Endocarditis may be caused by microorganisms or an immune response.

2. Pulmonary embolism refers to an obstruction of the pulmonary artery or one of its branches usually caused by an embolus from thrombosis in the lower extremities.

4. Pregnancy-induced hypertension (PIH) usually develops late in the second trimester or in the third trimester. The reason is unknown but it seems to be related to prenatal care, age, and parity.

Nursing Process: Planning
Client Need: Physiological Integrity

9 - 4 2

① The nurse will monitor the client for epigastric pain. Epigastric pain is a late sign in preeclampsia that may precede a seizure. The generalized edema that occurs in preeclampsia can stretch the liver capsule and cause subcapsular hemorrhage and severe epigastric pain.

2. Urinary output of 60 cc per hour is within normal limits.

3 and 4. Protein in the urine and facial edema are early signs of preeclampsia.

Nursing Process: Analyzing

Client Need: Physiological Integrity

9 - 4 3

③ The nurse understands that bromocriptine mesylate (Parlodel) was prescribed to inhibit secretion of the lactogenic hormone. Bromocriptine mesylate (Parlodel) is a dopamine receptor agonist that acts on receptors in the anterior lobe of the pituitary to inhibit secretion of prolactin and interfere with lactogenesis.

1. Bromocriptine mesylate does not directly affect sodium retention.

2. Bromocriptine mesylate does not suppress the production of chorionic gonadotropin. (Chorionic gonadotropins are present in the urine of pregnant women. The detection of gonadotropins serves as a basis for the pregnancy test.)

4. Bromocriptine mesylate does not diminish lochial flow (lochia refers to the discharge from the uterus of blood, mucus, and tissue during the puerperal period).

Nursing Process: Analyzing

Client Need: Health Promotion and Maintenance

9 - 4 4

③ To assess for contractions and for changes in the intensity of contractions, the nurse will place the hand flat on the abdomen over the fundus with the fingers apart and press lightly. Uterine contractions are initiated in the fundal portion of the uterus.

1, 2, and 4. Placing the hands on opposite sides of the abdomen, placing the heel of the hand on the abdomen, or placing the hand in the middle of the abdomen are incorrect methods of assessing for contractions and/or changes in the intensity of contractions.

Nursing Process: Assessing

Client Need: Health Promotion and Maintenance

9 - 4 5

② **A positive pregancy test is a probable sign that is objective because it is a definite indicator of pregnancy but does not constitute diagnosis or confirmation. Other probable signs include enlargement of the abdomen, changes in the cervix, and Braxton-Hicks contractions.**

1. Presumptive signs include menstrual suppression, nausea, vomiting, morning sickness, and pigmentation of the skin.

3 and 4. Positive signs and subjective signs are diagnostic and include fetal heart sound, fetal movement felt by the examiner, and roentgenogram outline of fetal skeleton.

Nursing Process: Assessing

Client Need: Physiological Integrity

9 - 4 6

① **A sudden increase in weight may be indicative of fluid retention. Recommended weight gain in the second and third trimester for a pregnant adolescent should be 0.4 kg (1 lb) per week. Because the client is an adolescent, she is at risk for developing preeclampsia. Edema is one of the primary signs of preeclampsia.**

2. 4½ lbs over a period of 4 weeks is not excessive.

3. A weight gain of 11 lbs in the second trimester is not excessive. This is a little less than 1 lb per week.

4. A weight gain of 14 lbs since onset of pregnancy is not excessive. This is about ½ lb per week.

Nursing Process: Analyzing

Client Need: Physiological Integrity

9 - 4 7

④ **The primary nursing diagnosis at this time would be altered tissue perfusion secondary to excessive blood loss. Hemorrhage can be life threatening and is therefore the first priority.**

1. The client is probably very concerned about her personal safety and the safety of the fetus. However, the first priority should be placed on interventions that will treat the profuse bleeding that could be life threatening.

2. If action isn't taken to treat the hemorrhage, the lives of both the mother and fetus could be lost.

3. There is no indication that the mucus plug has been lost.

Nursing Process: Analyzing

Client Need: Physiological Integrity

9 - 4 8

② **The nurse should evaluate the firmness and position of the fundus to prevent any further blood loss.**

1. The nurse will turn, cough, and deep breathe the client to prevent pneumonia and atelectasis, not to prevent excessive blood loss.

3. Administration of analgesics would help treat pain but would not affect blood loss.

4. The uterus should not be massaged routinely every 30 minutes; the client has had a cesarean section.

Nursing Process: Evaluating

Client Need: Health Promotion and Maintenance

9 - 4 9

③ **Couvade , Mitleiden, or "suffering along" are terms that describe the behavior of expectant fathers who manifest many of the physical symptoms, such as morning sickness, weight gain, abdominal pain, backache, and leg cramps, associated with their partner's pregnancy.**

1. It isn't the increase in the severity of symptoms that is associated with couvade but the fact that the fathers may experience the physical symptoms of pregnancy.

2. The fathers do not believe they are pregnant. However, they do experience the physical symptoms associated with pregnancy.

4. Telling a father that the physical symptoms he is experiencing will let him know "What happens to a pregnant woman," indicates a lack of concern on the part of the nurse and is not appropriate.

Nursing Process: Assessing

Client Need: Physiological Integrity

9 - 5 0

① **Following administration of an epidural, the nurse should assess the client for hypotension. Women who receive epidural anesthesia (an anesthetic agent placed in the epidural space) may experience relief of pain while being alert and relaxed during labor.**

2. Hypotension, not hypertension, should be anticipated following an epidural.

3. A headache is not associated with an epidural. However, headaches are associated with spinal taps.

4. Dyspnea is not associated with an epidural. However, injection of the epidural agent can cause respiratory paralysis and cardiovascular collapse.

Nursing Process: Assessing

Client Need: Health Promotion and Maintenance

Practice Test 10

Respiratory System and Acid-Base Imbalance

1 0 - 1

An elderly client admitted to the hospital because of "confusion" has been taking baking soda several times a day for the past week for an upset stomach. Which of the following laboratory results would you expect to see?

1. bicarbonate elevation
2. low pH
3. low sodium
4. potassium elevation

1 0 - 2

Your client had a lobectomy of the left lung. The client returns to the unit with a chest tube in place attached to a water-seal drainage. You observe fluid fluctuating in the chest tube with each respiration. Which interpretation of this observation is correct?

1. Oxygen is being lost through the client's chest tube with each respiration.
2. There is an air leak within the drainage system.
3. The apparatus is functioning properly.
4. Air is being drawn into the client's chest cavity.

1 0 - 3

To determine if a client with multidrug-resistant tuberculosis is no longer infectious, the client must:

1. remain afebrile for 5 days.
2. show a negative blood culture.
3. show negative daily sputum cultures for 3 consecutive days.
4. show a white blood cell count that is within normal limits.

1 0 - 4

An 82-year-old client has been admitted to the medical unit with a diagnosis of pneumonia. The client has an elevated temperature, respirations are rapid and shallow, and the client complains of chest pain. In order to decrease the client's chest pain, you would:

1. instruct the client to limit intake of air.
2. teach the client to increase the depth of respirations.
3. support the client's rib cage during coughing.
4. show the client how to relax the diaphragm.

10 - 5

A client with chronic obstructive pulmonary disease has been on prednisone for the past 2 years. The client is at risk for developing:

1. Cushing's syndrome.
2. Addison's disease.
3. Eaton-Lambert syndrome.
4. diabetes mellitus.

10 - 6

A client with chronic obstructive pulmonary disease is placed on a continuous aminophylline drip. The nurse knows that aminophylline may:

1. strengthen the heartbeat.
2. increase the heart rate.
3. dilate the coronary arteries.
4. decrease myocardial oxygen demand.

10 - 7

A client has had a bronchoscopy. Which of the following nursing observations would indicate possible complications?

1. The client coughs up small amounts of blood-tinged sputum.
2. The client complains of difficulty in breathing.
3. The client is very hoarse when speaking.
4. The client complains of a sore throat when swallowing.

10 - 8

After a bronchoscopy, your client experiences the following problems. Which would indicate a need for further observation?

1. cough
2. dry mouth
3. sore throat
4. dyspnea

10-9

A client with chronic obstructive pulmonary disease enters the clinic experiencing shortness of breath, nausea, and dizziness. To assess the client's level of hypoxia, the nurse will:

1. obtain a throat culture.
2. obtain a sputum collection.
3. utilize an incentive spirometer.
4. utilize a pulse oximetry.

10-10

The nursing diagnosis, activity intolerance related to decreased oxygenation, is established for a client. To promote activity tolerance in the client, the nurse will plan to:

1. have the client decide which activities will be completed for the day.
2. complete all care at one time to avoid disturbing the client later.
3. space nursing activities to allow the client frequent rest periods.
4. suggest ways in which the client can participate in performing care.

10-11

A 3-year-old is admitted to the hospital with a medical diagnosis of laryngotracheobronchitis. A mist tent with oxygen has been prescribed. Because the client is restless and crying, the nurse is unable to obtain an accurate respiration rate. Which action should the nurse take?

1. Ask another staff member to count the client's respirations.
2. Record an approximate respiratory rate.
3. Wait until the client is quiet before counting respirations.
4. Average the client's respirations per minute after taking them for 3 minutes.

10-12

A client who experiences severe asthma may develop life-threatening acid-base disturbances. Which of the following blood gas results would be most indicative of pending respiratory failure?

1. PO_2 of 90 mmHg
2. pH of 7.40
3. PCO_2 of 65 mmHg
4. O_2 saturation of 92%

10-13

The hallmark of chronic bronchitis is:

1. a daily productive cough.
2. dyspnea.
3. cyanosis.
4. right ventricular failure.

10-14

The nurse observes a client with tuberculosis putting a soiled disposable tissue in an ashtray. Which response would be appropriate for the nurse to make?

1. "Let me get you a disposable bag for your used tissue."
2. "Let me get you an emesis basin to dispose of your used tissue."
3. "Did you receive instructions about disposal of soiled tissues?"
4. "Can I help you dispose of your soiled tissue?"

10-15

Oxygen is best delivered to the hypoxic client during meals by:

1. endotracheal tube.
2. face mask.
3. face tent.
4. nasal cannula.

10-16

The nurse begins resuscitation on a 4-year-old who has stopped breathing. To administer effective breaths for the child, the nurse should:

1. pinch off the child's nares and hyperextend the child's neck.
2. pinch off the child's nares and slightly extend the child's neck.
3. lift the child's jaw and breathe into the child's nares.
4. encircle and breathe into the mouth and nares of the child.

10-17

A client has a chest tube attached to a water-seal drainage. Which of the following nursing measures is most important in preventing respiratory complications?

1. securing the tubing above the level of the incision
2. reinforcing the dressing over the insertion site
3. sealing the air vent on the suction control chamber of the drainage system
4. keeping the water-seal drainage system near the floor

10-18

A client will receive atropine 0.4 mg intramuscularly 30 minutes before surgery. The nurse knows the purpose of this medication is to:

1. facilitate the effects of anesthesia.
2. prevent postoperative dehydration.
3. improve smooth muscle tone and prevent hemorrhage.
4. reduce oral and respiratory secretions during surgery.

10-19

A client who has adrenal insufficiency is to receive fludrocortisone acetate 0.1 mg by mouth. As you prepare to give this medicine, your client complains of dyspnea. You observe bilateral moist crackles in the lungs and a new S_3. You will:

1. give the dose as prescribed.
2. give the dose intravenously.
3. give twice the prescribed dose.
4. hold the dose and notify the physician.

10-20

Your 67-year-old client collapses while ambulating in the hall. The client is not breathing and does not have a palpable pulse. CPR is initiated. As soon as the client is connected to the monitor/defibrillator, you see that the EKG shows ventricular fibrillation. You know that the client requires defibrillation, with a current dosage beginning at:

1. 2 joules.
2. 20 joules.
3. 200 joules.
4. 2000 joules.

10-21

Your client will have chest tubes attached to a water-seal drainage following surgery. During preoperative teaching, you will inform the client that the purpose of chest tubes is to:

1. allow for the removal of fluid and air.
2. make deep breathing and coughing easier.
3. prevent rapid reexpansion of the lung.
4. control internal hemorrhage.

10-22

Upon admittance to your intensive care unit, a client's laboratory work is serum glucose = 898 mg/dL, arterial blood pH = 7.10, arterial blood HCO_3 = 11 mEq/L, and arterial blood PCO_2 = 37 mmHg. You anticipate the need to administer, in addition to insulin, the following treatment:

1. hetastarch 500 intravenously stat.
2. immediate intubation and hyperinflation to combat respiratory acidosis.
3. 1 unit of packed red blood cells given stat.
4. sodium bicarbonate infusion to combat metabolic acidosis.

10-23

An agitated client has diazepam prescribed, 5 mg intravenously every 2 hours as needed. After administering a dose, you notice that the client's respiratory rate has dropped from 20 breaths per min to 6 breaths per min. You know to administer:

1. fentanyl citrate.
2. fluorouracil.
3. fluconazole.
4. flumazenil.

10-24

This is your client's first postoperative day following a pneumonectomy. For evening nourishment, several beverages will be available. Which one will facilitate wound healing the best?

1. tomato juice
2. apple juice
3. orange juice
4. grapefruit juice

10-25

A client has bronchiectasis. In evaluating the effects of a prescribed expectorant, the nurse will anticipate:

1. cough suppression.
2. bronchial dilation.
3. reduced viscosity of respiratory secretions.
4. decreased production of respiratory secretions.

10-26

A fullterm newborn is 1-day postoperative after a successful repair of a tracheo-esophageal fistula. The postoperative plan of care will include:

1. minimizing handling and stimulation.
2. gentle suctioning of oral secretions hourly.
3. frequent respiratory and abdominal assessment.
4. gastrostomy feedings every 2 to 3 hours.

10-27

Clients planning to use Nicoderm should be advised to:

1. start with a low dose and gradually increase the dosage.
2. change the patch weekly.
3. anticipate a lifetime of patch use.
4. rotate patch sites daily.

10-28

A mist tent has been prescribed for a 2-year-old client with bacterial pneumonia. When the mother of the client visits, she tells the nurse, "I just put my hand in the tent and my child's clothing is damp." Which action should the nurse take in response to the mother's comments?

1. Report the mother's conversation to the nurse in charge.
2. Encourage the client to drink fluids to replace those that were lost.
3. Take the client's body temperature and compare it with previous body temperatures.
4. Explain the purpose of humidity to the mother.

1 0 - 2 9

Your client is experiencing metabolic acidosis. A compensatory mechanism seen in clients experiencing metabolic acidosis is:

1. a deep, gasping type of respiration.
2. a marked, sustained inspiratory effort.
3. several short breaths followed by long irregular periods of apnea.
4. periods of apnea lasting 10 to 60 seconds followed by gradually increasing depth and frequency of respirations.

1 0 - 3 0

The nurse delivers oxygen by hood to a preterm neonate. Which arterial blood gas indicates the intervention has been most effective?

1. pH 7.30, PCO_2 45, PO_2 45
2. pH 7.28, PCO_2 50, PO_2 40
3. pH 7.37, PCO_2 40, PO_2 80
4. pH 7.42, PCO_2 22, PO_2 100

1 0 - 3 1

A client with chest pain arrives at your unit. Prescriptions read "Oxygen 2 to 4 liters per minute." There is history of chronic obstructive pulmonary disease. In addition to the oxygen saturation level, what other data must be considered when choosing an oxygen dosage?

1. hemoglobin
2. serum potassium
3. serum chloride
4. height

1 0 - 3 2

Which of the following symptoms would be the best indicator of a tension pneumothorax?

1. spitting up blood
2. sucking sounds made on inspiration
3. collapsed and flat-looking neck veins
4. deviation of the trachea

10-33

Your client had a radical neck dissection. In the immediate postoperative period, you detect the presence of stridor. You understand the most probable cause of stridor is:

1. laryngeal obstruction.
2. respiratory insufficiency.
3. mediastinal shifting.
4. congestive heart failure.

10-34

A client was admitted to the Emergency Department following a car accident. You note paradoxical movement of the chest wall and respiratory distress. What do you suspect is causing this?

1. pneumonia
2. flail chest
3. pneumothorax
4. cardiac tamponade

10-35

Your asthmatic client is being discharged home with the prescription "Beclomethasone dipropionate 2 puffs qid with spacer." When asked by your client about the use of this inhaler during status asthmaticus, you reply:

1. "It is for use during status asthmaticus; take 4 puffs."
2. "It is for use during status asthmaticus; remove the spacer prior to dosing."
3. "Status asthmaticus will never happen again."
4. "This is not to treat status asthmaticus."

10-36

Your client is intubated and on mechanical ventilation. Pancuronium bromide has been prescribed. You know that this medication:

1. may cause marked bradycardia.
2. may be given even after your client is off of the ventilator.
3. is an analgesic with hypnotic effect.
4. should be given with sedation or analgesia.

10-37

You are concerned that your client may be developing adult respiratory distress syndrome following a motor vehicle accident. What early manifestations of adult respiratory distress syndrome do you need to assess at this time?

1. dyspnea and tachypnea
2. cyanosis and apprehension
3. hemoptysis
4. diffuse crackles and rhonchi

10-38

A client has developed acute renal failure following a course of antibiotic therapy with the aminoglycoside tobramycin. Daily laboratory tests have been prescribed to monitor the progression of the disease. Which of the following arterial blood gas profiles is indicative of renal acidosis?

1. pH 7.35, PaO_2 95, $PaCO_2$ 35, HCO_3 20
2. pH 7.36, PaO_2 98, $PaCO_2$ 32, HCO_3 23
3. pH 7.40, PaO_2 78, $PaCO_2$ 50, HCO_3 38
4. pH 7.15, PaO_2 99, $PaCO_2$ 38, HCO_3 8

10-39

A client has been diagnosed with chronic obstructive pulmonary lung disease. Coughing has become increasingly productive. The sputum is thick and yellowish in color. The client is being treated with theophylline 100 mg po, qid. Theophylline is given to:

1. relieve bronchospasm.
2. decrease sputum production.
3. suppress coughing.
4. treat respiratory infection.

10-40

A client is experiencing Kussmaul respirations. These respirations:

1. act as a distraction for the client during painful episodes.
2. help the body rid itself of excess fluids.
3. enhance circulation by increased chest wall movement.
4. serve as a secondary defense in an attempt to get rid of hydrogen ions.

10-41

In addition to dehydration, elderly persons who experience prolonged diarrhea are at risk for which of the following disturbances?

1. hyperkalemia
2. respiratory acidosis
3. hypernatremia
4. metabolic acidosis

10-42

A client with multiple drug-resistant tuberculosis has been admitted to your unit. What do you expect your assessment to reveal?

1. crackles, cyanosis, and fever
2. fever, weight loss, and night sweats
3. sudden chest pain, hemoptysis, and tachycardia
4. nausea, diaphoresis, and severe chest pain

10-43

A client is admitted to the Emergency Department with multiple knife wounds to the chest. The knife is still in the client's chest. What should you do?

1. remove the knife
2. cleanse the chest wounds with saline
3. seal open chest wounds with an airtight dressing
4. place the client in a supine position

10-44

Two hours ago, a client's oxygen concentration was decreased to 40% oxygen by mask. The client's arterial oxygen pressure value also decreased by 20% to 50 mm Hg. Which of the following would you do initially?

1. Do nothing; the drop in arterial oxygen pressure is an expected outcome.
2. Increase the oxygen concentration to 60%.
3. Assess the client's situation and inform the physician of the changes.
4. Closely monitor the client's condition.

10-45

A client is receiving aminophylline to treat pulmonary emphysema that has been complicated by an upper respiratory infection. To evaluate the effectiveness of this drug, the nurse should monitor the:

1. amount and color of secretions.
2. rate and rhythm of respirations.
3. pattern of temperature elevations.
4. expansion of the chest cavity.

10-46

A client has chest tubes and needs to be transported to radiation therapy for treatment. Which of the following nursing actions is appropriate to provide safety during transport?

1. Keep the water-seal unit close to the client by taping it to the abdominal area.
2. Clamp the chest tube before disconnecting it from the water-seal unit.
3. Attach the rubber-tipped forceps to the client's gown before transport.
4. Instruct the client to take deep breaths should the chest tube become dislodged.

10-47

A client with amyotrophic lateral sclerosis is brought to the Emergency Department in respiratory arrest. The best method to use when administering oxygen to this client would be by:

1. positive pressure ventilation.
2. nasal cannula.
3. face mask.
4. oxygen tent.

10-48

A client has had a resection of the right lung. A chest tube has been inserted and the client is also receiving oxygen. In addition to administering the prescribed analgesic, which of the following actions should the nurse take that would provide the most comfort for the client while coughing and deep breathing?

1. administering analgesics and splinting the chest with a pillow
2. elevating the head of the bed
3. clamping the chest tube
4. removing the oxygen temporarily

1 0 - 4 9

A client is receiving oxygen therapy by face mask. Which measures should the nurse include in the plan of care?

1. taking the body temperature rectally
2. giving a complete bed bath
3. encouraging additional fluids
4. assisting with coughing and deep-breathing exercises.

1 0 - 5 0

A client with chronic obstructive pulmonary disease is in respiratory distress. To facilitate breathing, the nurse will place the client in which position?

1. supine and dorsal recumbent
2. dorsal with the head down and the feet elevated
3. upright at 90 degrees
4. semi-prone on the left side with right knee drawn up toward the chest

Practice Test 10

Answers, Rationales, and Explanations

10-1

① **You will expect to see a bicarbonate elevation. Baking soda or sodium bicarbonate is used by some individuals as a home remedy for indigestion. This may, however, cause severe acid-base disturbances and may also cause an elevation in the serum bicarbonate level and a subsequent metabolic alkalosis.**

2 and 3. The nurse would anticipate a pH elevation with the ingestion of sodium bicarbonate and its subsequent metabolic alkalosis as well as an increase in serum sodium.

4. The serum potassium would not be immediately or directly affected at this time.

Nursing Process: Evaluating
Client Need: Physiological Integrity

10-2

③ **You would understand that the apparatus is functioning properly. If fluctuations do not occur, something is plugging the tubing or the lung has reinflated.**

1. Oxygen is not being lost through the client's chest tube with each respiration. The fluctuation indicates proper functioning. The purpose of chest tubes is to drain fluid and air from the pleural space and reestablish negative pressure. The fact that the fluid in the chest tube is fluctuating indicates the water-seal drainage is functioning properly.

2. If there is an air leak within the drainage system, the nurse would observe a continuous bubbling (not intermittent) in the water-seal. This must be corrected by locating the source of the leak and repairing it.

4. If air was being drawn into the client's chest cavity, the nurse would observe signs and symptoms of a collapsed lung or mediastinal shift such as dyspnea, anxiety, diaphoresis, and tachycardia.

Nursing Process: Evaluating
Client Need: Physiological Integrity

10-3

③ **Sputum cultures on 3 consecutive mornings must be negative for the tubercular bacillus for a client to be considered no longer infectious.**

1, 2, and 4. Remaining afebrile for 5 days, showing a negative blood culture, and showing a white blood cell count that is within normal limits are not tests that determine if clients with multidrug-resistant tuberculosis are no longer infectious. The sputum cultures must be negative for 3 consecutive days.

Nursing Process: Evaluating
Client Need: Physiological Integrity

10 - 4

③ **Supporting the rib cage during coughing will diminish pain and at the same time facilitate increased diaphragmatic movement.**

1. Instructing the client to limit intake of air is contraindicated.

2. Telling the client to increase the depth of respirations will help treat the pneumonia. However, this will not directly relieve the chest pain.

4. Showing the client how to relax the diaphragm will not relieve the pain.

Nursing Process: Implementing
Client Need: Health Promotion and Maintenance

10 - 5

① **The client is at risk for developing Cushing's syndrome due to long-term steroid use. This is the most frequent cause of Cushing's syndrome seen in clinical practice.**

2. Addison's disease occurs when there is an inadequate amount of cortisol secreted.

3. Eaton-Lambert syndrome is an autoimmune disorder caused by impaired presynaptic release of acetycholine at nerve synapses.

4. Steroids do alter carbohydrate metabolism; however, just taking steroids does not increase the risk of developing diabetes unless the client is already predisposed to developing it.

Nursing Process: Analyzing
Client Need: Physiological Integrity

10 - 6

② **The nurse knows that aminophylline increases the heart rate as well as dilating the bronchi. Tachycardia is a frequent side effect experienced by clients receiving this medication.**

1. Digitalis preparations frequently strengthen the heartbeat.

3. Nitrates dilate the coronary arteries.

4. Calcium channel-blockers will decrease the myocardial oxygen demand.

Nursing Process: Analyzing
Client Need: Health Promotion and Maintenance

10-7

② **Difficulty in breathing (dyspnea) would indicate a possible complication associated with a bronchoscopic examination. A serious complication following a bronchoscopy would be swelling due to the trauma of the procedure. The first symptom the client would experience is difficulty in breathing. Other complications associated with a bronchoscopic examination include reaction to local anesthesia, aspiration, bronchospasm, pneumothorax, hemorrhage, and perforation.**

1. Coughing up small amounts of blood-tinged sputum could occur because of irritation to the mucous membranes during the procedure. This would not be considered a complication.

3. Bronchoscopy is the direct visual inspection of the larynx, trachea, and bronchi; therefore, hoarseness could occur and would not be considered a complication.

4. A sore throat is not unusual because of the irritating effects of the examination.

Nursing Process: Assessing
Client Need: Physiological Integrity

10-8

④ **Signs of difficult breathing would indicate a need for further observation. After a bronchoscopy, a client should be observed closely for signs and symptoms of laryngospasm or laryngeal edema that result in dyspnea (difficult breathing). If impaired respirations occur, immediate interventions are necessary, i.e., intubation.**

1, 2, and 3. Coughing, dry mouth, and sore throat are not unusual following a bronchoscopy and would not be indicators of further problems.

Nursing Process: Evaluating
Client Need: Physiological Integrity

10-9

④ **To assess the client's level of hypoxia, the nurse will use a pulse oximetry. A pulse oximetry is a noninvasive device that measures a client's arterial blood oxygen saturation and can detect hypoxemia before clinical signs appear.**

1. A throat culture is used to assess the presence of disease-producing microorganisms.

2. A sputum collection is obtained to identify a specific microorganism and its drug sensitivities.

3. An incentive spirometer is a device that gradually increases air flow into the lungs. It does not assess for hypoxia.

Nursing Process: Assessing
Client Need: Physiological Integrity

10-10

③ **To promote activity tolerance in the client, the nurse will space nursing activities. Spacing activities diminishes the amount of oxygen needed at any one time and allows the oxygen reserves to be built up during periods of rest.**

1. Having the client decide which activities will be completed each day will not affect oxygen reserves.

2. Completing all care at one time would deplete oxygen reserves and would be contraindicated.

4. There are energy-efficient methods that could be helpful for clients to learn in performing their care. However, it is the spacing of activities that allows for build-up of oxygen reserves.

Nursing Process: Planning
Client Need: Physiological Integrity

10-11

③ **The nurse should postpone assessing respirations until the child becomes quiet. Every effort should be made to avoid further aggravation of the child's respiratory distress.**

1. Having another staff member attempt to count the child's respirations may upset the child further and is not recommended.

2 and 4. The child has a respiratory condition. Respirations should be counted for 1 full minute, not estimated or averaged.

Nursing Process: Evaluating
Client Need: Physiological Integrity

10-12

③ **A PCO_2 of 65 mmHg is indicative of impending respiratory failure. The normal pressure exerted by carbon dioxide gas in arterial blood (the PCO_2) is 38 to 44 mmHg. Pressures over 50 mmHg suggest there is excess PCO_2 in the blood and acidosis is developing. Respiratory failure is a grave potential should this occur.**

1, 2, and 4. These values are all within the normal ranges. The pressure exerted by oxygen (PO_2) in arterial blood is 80 to 105 mmHg, the normal pH is between 7.35 to 7.45, and the normal O_2 saturation is > 90%.

Nursing Process: Analyzing
Client Need: Physiological Integrity

10-13

① **The hallmark of chronic bronchitis is a daily productive cough that lasts about 3 months out of the year for 2 consecutive years.**

2, 3, and 4. Chronic bronchitis progresses to dyspnea, cyanosis, and right ventricular failure.

Nursing Process: Assessing
Client Need: Physiological Integrity

10-14

① **It would be appropriate for the nurse to see that the client's soiled tissue is placed in a disposable bag. Clients with tuberculosis should place all soiled tissues into a disposable bag. Sputum-laden tissues should be confined to a closed container that can be disposed of in institutional incinerators. Proper handling of sputum prevents the organisms from becoming airborne.**

2. Placing soiled tissues in an open emesis basin exposes others to the tubercle bacillus.

3. Assessing what the client knows concerning the disposal of contaminated materials should come after the soiled tissue has been disposed of properly.

4. Asking a client if you can help with the disposal of a soiled tissue might be answered in the negative.

Nursing Process: Implementing
Client Need: Safe, Effective Care Environment

10-15

④ **Oxygen is best delivered to the hypoxic client during meals by nasal cannula. A prong is placed into each nostril that delivers low-flow oxygen without a need for restricted mouth movement. Clients may talk, drink, and eat while receiving oxygen by nasal cannula without interrupting the oxygen flow.**

1. Endotracheal tubes are taped in place until they are no longer needed to assist ventilation and clients are not fed through the mouth.

2 and 3. Face masks and tents must be removed prior to eating.

Nursing Process: Implementing
Client Need: Safe, Effective Care Environment

10-16

② **To administer effective breaths for a 4-year-old child, the nurse will pinch off the child's nares and slightly extend the child's neck.**

1. A child's head should not be hyperextended during resuscitation because the trachea is soft and hyperextension could compress it.

3 and 4. Breathing into the nose (nares) and mouth simultaneously is appropriate only for infants.

Nursing Process: Implementing
Client Need: Physiological Integrity

10-17

④ **Keeping the water-seal drainage system near the floor is the most important nursing measure the nurse can take to prevent respiratory complications. Maintaining the water-seal drainage system below the client's chest will prevent backflow of fluid and air into the client's pleural cavity.**

1. Securing the tubing above the level of the incision will cause a backflow of air and fluid into the pleural cavity.

2. The dressing should not be reinforced unless there is a leak at the insertion site.

3. Water-seal drainage must have an air vent to provide an escape route for air passing through the water seal from the pleural space.

Nursing Process: Implementing
Client Need: Physiological Integrity

10-18

④ **The purpose for administering atropine preoperatively is to prevent aspiration by reducing oral and respiratory secretions. Atropine is an anticholinergic that, when given properly, reduces oral and respiratory secretions.**

1. A frequent side effect of atropine is drowsiness. However, drowsiness is not an expected outcome and is not administered to produce drowsiness or to facilitate the effects of anesthesia.

2. Atropine does not affect hydration nor does it contribute to dehydration postoperatively.

3. Atropine does not affect smooth muscle tone or prevent hemorrhage.

Nursing Process: Evaluating
Client Need: Safe, Effective Care Environment

10-19

④ **You will hold the dose of fludrocortisone acetate (Florinef) and notify the physician if you auscultate bilateral moist crackles in the lungs and a new S$_3$ sound. Florinef may cause sodium and water retention and is not to be given to those who manifest signs of pulmonary edema such as dyspnea and crackles.**

1. The fludrocortisone acetate is contraindicated in clients suspected of pulmonary edema.
2. The route has been prescribed (po); however, the client has bilateral moist crackles and an S$_3$ sound. You would withhold the medication.
3. No amount of fludrocortisone acetate should be administered to this client because of bilateral crackles and the S$_3$ sound. The dosage should be withheld and the physician notified of the client's condition.

Nursing Process: Implementing
Client Need: Health Promotion and Maintenance

10-20

③ **Two hundred joules is the recommended initial defibrillation dosage for an adult experiencing ventricular fibrillation.**

1. Two joules is a neonate dosage.
2. Twenty joules is a pediatric dosage.
4. Two thousand joules is an overdose and unobtainable on a defibrillator.

Nursing Process: Evaluating
Client Need: Physiological Integrity

10-21

① **The nurse will inform the preoperative client that the purpose of chest tube insertion into the pleural space is to allow for the drainage of fluid and air and to reestablish negative pressure.**

2. Deep breathing and coughing will become easier once fluid and air have been removed from the pleural space and negative pressure has been reestablished.
3. The lungs will expand as the fluid and air are removed from the pleural space.
4. Chest tubes do not have an impact on internal hemorrhage. However, a rising fluid level in the collection chamber, a drop in blood pressure, and rapid pulse are indicators of hemorrhage.

Nursing Process: Implementing
Client Need: Safe, Effective Care Environment

10-22

④ **In addition to the insulin, the client should receive a sodium bicarbonate infusion to combat metabolic acidosis. This laboratory work suggests metabolic acidosis because a pH of 7.10 is less than the normal range of 7.35 to 7.45. The bicarbonate level (HCO₃) is low also, at 11 mEq/L; the normal is 22 to 26 mEq/L. This combination of abnormals indicates a metabolic acidosis, the treatment for which is empirically sodium bicarbonate, an alkalyzing agent.**

1. There is no evidence that fluid volume replacement is needed. Hetastarch (Hespan) is a volume expander usually used for shock due to burns, hemorrhage, sepsis, and trauma.

2. The client is in metabolic acidosis, not respiratory acidosis.

3. There is no indication that the hemoglobin is low. Therefore, there is no need for packed red blood cells.

Nursing Process: Analyzing
Client Need: Physiological Integrity

10-23

④ **You will administer flumazenil. Flumazenil (Romazicon) is a benzodiazepine antagonist whose competitive inhibition of the receptor sites blocks the action of benzodiazepines. In this instance, the respiratory depression due to diazepam (Valium) administration would be corrected.**

1. Fentanyl citrate is an anesthetic agent.

2. Fluorouracil is an antineoplastic agent.

3. Fluconazole is an antifungal agent.

Nursing Process: Implementing
Client Need: Physiological Integrity

10-24

③ **Orange juice facilitates wound healing better than apple, tomato, or grapefruit juice. Orange juice contains high amounts of vitamin C. Vitamin C helps to form collagen, which plays an important role in wound healing.**

1. Tomato juice is higher in vitamin C than apple juice but not as high as orange and grapefruit.

2. Apple juice has the least amount of vitamin C compared to tomato, orange, or grapefruit.

4. Grapefruit juice has the second highest amount of vitamin C compared to orange, tomato, or apple juice.

Nursing Process: Implementing
Client Need: Physiological Integrity

10-25

③ The nurse will anticipate an expectorant (mucokinetic agent) to improve the removal of respiratory secretions by thinning and decreasing the viscosity of the secretions in the client experiencing bronchiectasis.

1. Antitussives are administered to provide symptomatic relief of coughing by suppressing the cough reflex.

2. Bronchodilators are administered to reverse airway obstruction and prevent bronchospasm.

4. Anticholinergics decrease production of respiratory and oral secretions.

Nursing Process: Evaluating
Client Need: Physiological Integrity

10-26

③ Frequent respiratory and abdominal assessment of the infant with a repair of a tracheoesophageal fistula is necessary since it is very likely that the infant aspirated prior to surgery and because the chest cavity was opened during surgery. Abdominal assessment would also verify the return of peristalsis and the presence of distension associated with peritonitis.

1. Periodic stimulation will encourage deep breathing and reinflation of the infant's lungs, and therefore should not be minimized.

2. Oral secretions should not need suctioning since they are not copious and can be effectively swallowed.

4. Intravenous feeding can be used for several days to allow for initial healing of the esophageal repair.

Nursing Process: Implementing
Client Need: Physiological Integrity

10-27

④ Clients planning to use Nicoderm should be advised to rotate patch sites daily. Nicotine transdermal (Nicoderm) is a graduated nicotine patch designed to relieve withdrawal symptoms from tobacco cessation. Because the patches contain nicotine, they may be irritating to the skin and the sites should be rotated daily.

1. Administration of Nicoderm starts with a higher dosage and then the dosage is gradually decreased.

2. The Nicoderm patches should be changed daily, not weekly.

3. Nicoderm patches are designed to be used for 2 to 3 months and are then discontinued.

Nursing Process: Implementing
Client Need: Physiological Integrity

10-28

④ **The nurse will explain to the mother that the function of the mist tent is to generate high humidity, which will help to liquefy respiratory secretions. The dampness on the child's clothing is due to condensation and is not harmful.**

1. There is no need to report the mother's conversation since the dampness of the child's clothing is an expected consequence of the humidity.

2 and 3. The dampness of the child's clothing is due to the humidity produced by the tent, not perspiration or an elevation of the child's body temperature.

Nursing Process: Implementing
Client Need: Physiological Integrity

10-29

① **A compensatory mechanism seen in clients experiencing metabolic acidosis is a deep, gasping type of respiration called Kussmaul breathing. Kussmaul breathing is a compensating mechanism present in clients experiencing metabolic acidosis and renal failure. Kussmaul breathing is called air hunger and exceeds 20 breaths per minute.**

2. Apneustic breathing is a marked, sustained respiratory effort associated with central nervous system disorders.

3. Biot's respirations are shallow breaths with apnea seen in clients with increased intracranial pressure.

4. Cheyne-Stokes respirations are rhythmic waxing and waning, deep to shallow temporary apnea. This type of respiration is pathological in the adult but is normal in children.

Nursing Process: Analyzing
Client Need: Physiological Integrity

10-30

③ **Arterial blood gases showing a pH of 7.37, a PCO_2 of 40, and a PO_2 of 80 indicate the interventions have been effective. A pH of 7.37 is within the normal limits of 7.35 to 7.45. A partial pressure of carbon dioxide (PCO_2) of 40 is within the normal limits of 35 to 45 mmHg. A partial pressure of oxygen (PO_2) of 80 is within the normal limits of 75 to 95 mmHg.**

1. pH 7.30, PCO_2 45, PO_2 45 = pH too low, PCO_2 almost too high, and PO_2 too low.
2. pH 7.28, PCO_2 50, PO_2 40 = Respiratory acidosis.
4. pH 7.42, PCO_2 22, PO_2 100 = Respiratory alkalosis.

Nursing Process: Evaluating
Client Need: Physiological Integrity

10-31

① **In addition to the oxygen saturation level, other data that need to be considered when choosing an oxygen dosage is hemoglobin. Oxygen is carried by hemoglobin; hemoglobin is the part of the blood to which oxygen binds and is transported. A person with low hemoglobin has little capacity for oxygen transport. Supplemental oxygen would be indicated to maximize available oxygen transport.**

2, 3, and 4. Serum potassium, serum chloride, and a client's height have little bearing on oxygen levels.

Nursing Process: Evaluating
Client Need: Health Promotion and Maintenance

10-32

④ **Deviation of the trachea would suggest a tension pneumothorax. Tension pneumothorax is caused by an injury that perforates the chest wall or a lacerated lung that allows air to enter the pleural space. The air becomes trapped and builds up pressure, which causes the lung on the injured side to collapse. When the lung collapses, mediastinum shifting to the other side of the body occurs.**

1. Spitting up blood (hemoptysis) is indicative of a pulmonary embolism.
2. Sucking sounds made on inspiration are indicative of an open pneumothorax caused by an opening in the chest large enough to allow air to pass in and out freely during respirations.
3. Collapsed and flat-looking neck veins are indicative of dehydration.

Nursing Process: Assessing
Client Need: Safe, Effective Care Environment

10-33

① **The most probable cause of stridor following a radical neck dissection is laryngeal obstruction. Laryngeal stridor is identified upon auscultation of the trachea with a stethoscope. A coarse, high-pitched sound can be heard on inspiration. The most probable cause of stridor following a radical neck dissection is edema of the larynx. The surgeon should be notified immediately to prevent complete airway obstruction.**

2. Respiratory insufficiency is a condition in which respirations are not adequate to meet the body's need for oxygen following physical activity. Respiratory insufficiency is not associated with stridor.

3. Mediastinal shifting occurs in response to severe trauma to the chest that traps air in the pleural space (tension pneumothorax). As the volume of trapped air increases, the lung collapses and organs shift to the opposite side of the chest. Symptoms include displacement of the trachea, dyspnea, cyanosis, and displacement of neck veins. Mediastinal shift is not associated with stridor.

4. Congestive heart failure (CHF) occurs when the heart is unable to meet the body's need for oxygen and abnormal retention of sodium and water accumulates in the body. CHF is not a cause of stridor.

Nursing Process: Assessing
Client Need: Physiological Integrity

10-34

② **You will suspect flail chest. Flail chest is manifested by paradoxical movement of the chest wall and respiratory distress. The usual cause is fractured ribs, causing loss of chest wall stability. The flail segment will move paradoxically in with inspiration and out with expiration.**

1. Clinical manifestations of pneumonia include fever, chills, productive cough, and pleuritic chest pain.

3. Clinical manifestations of pneumothorax include diminished breath sounds on the injured side.

4. Clinical manifestations of cardiac tamponade are muffled and distant heart sounds, decreased blood pressure or pulse, steadily increasing central venous pressure, and possible distension of neck veins.

Nursing Process: Analyzing
Client Need: Physiological Integrity

10-35

④ **The nurse will tell the client that beclomethasone dipropionate does not treat status asthmaticus. Beclomethasone dipropionate is not a bronchodilator but a steroid, and the full therapeutic anti-inflammatory action may take days.**

1. Beclomethasone dipropionate medication doesn't treat status asthmaticus.

2. Beclomethasone dipropionate medication doesn't treat status asthmaticus, and the spacer's function is to ensure accurate dosing.

3. Status asthmaticus is a risk for every asthmatic client.

Nursing Process: Implementing
Client Need: Physiological Integrity

10-36

④ **You know that pancuronium should be given with sedation or analgesia. This paralytic agent doesn't affect pain sensation or anxiety levels and is very stressful to the client if given independently.**

1. Pancuronium bromide commonly causes tachycardia, not bradycardia.

2. Pancuronium bromide is a neuromuscular blocker.

3. Pancuronium bromide does not affect pain threshold or consciousness.

Nursing Process: Implementing
Client Need: Physiological Integrity

10-37

① **Early manifestations of adult respiratory distress syndrome (ARDS) are dyspnea and tachypnea. Other manifestations include cough and restlessness. ARDS is a sudden, progressive disorder consisting of pulmonary edema of noncardiac origin, severe dyspnea, hypoxemia, reduced lung compliance, and diffuse pulmonary infiltrates.**

2. Cyanosis and apprehension are later manifestations of ARDS.

3. Hemoptysis refers to blood-tinged or bloody sputum. True hemoptysis is bright red and frothy, indicating bleeding in the respiratory tract.

4. Diffuse crackles (rales) and rhonchi are later manifestations of ARDS.

Nursing Process: Analyzing
Client Need: Physiological Integrity

1 0 - 3 8

④ **Arterial blood gases showing a pH of 7.15, a PaO$_2$ of 99, a PaCO$_2$ of 38, and a HCO$_3$ of 8 are indicators of renal acidosis. A pH of<7.35 generally indicates an acidosis, as is seen here. Low bicarbonate levels <22 mEq/L generally indicate that the acidosis is metabolic in origin, especially since the respiratory parameter (the PaCO$_2$) is normal.**

1. This profile shows parameters are within normal range.

2. This profile suggest hyperventilation; all parameters are within normal range except the PaCO$_2$ (normal 35 to 45 tops).

3. This profile suggests compensated respiratory acidosis: normal pH value with PaCO$_2$ retention and low PaCO$_2$ (hypoventilation). The high HCO$_3$ value is due to renal compensation.

Nursing Process: Evaluating

Client Need: Health Promotion and Maintenance

1 0 - 3 9

① **Theophylline (Theo-dur) is given to relieve bronchospasm. By relieving bronchospasm, theophylline allays airway obstruction.**

2. Theophylline does not decrease sputum production.

3. Theophylline does not suppress coughing.

4. Theophylline does not treat respiratory infections.

Nursing Process: Implementing

Client Need: Physiological Integrity

1 0 - 4 0

④ **Kussmaul respirations serve as a secondary defense mechanism in which the body attempts to rid itself of excess hydrogen ions (H$^+$) that have accumulated due to conditions such as diabetic ketoacidosis. Kussmaul respirations are deep and often rapid respirations that are present during times of metabolic acidosis.**

1. Clients experiencing Kussmaul respirations are not in pain.

2. The purpose of Kussmaul respirations is to rid the body of excessive hydrogen ions.

3. Kussmaul respirations do increase chest wall movement but this is not the primary function of these respirations.

Nursing Process: Evaluating

Client Need: Physiological Integrity

10-41

④ Elderly persons who experience prolonged diarrhea are at risk for metabolic acidosis. Bicarbonate is housed in gastrointestinal secretions. When copious amounts of these secretions are lost, such as through prolonged diarrhea, bicarbonate ions are lost. This loss affects the blood pH in an increase in the overall concentration of hydrogen ions, thus a decrease in pH, or acidosis.

1, 2, and 3. Potassium and sodium are excreted in diarrhea, thus placing these clients at risk for hypokalemia and hyponatremia, not hyperkalemia and hypernatremia. This also causes a metabolic, not respiratory, acidosis, although respiratory compensation will eventually occur.

Nursing Process: Analyzing
Client Need: Physiological Integrity

10-42

② The nurse would expect an assessment of a client experiencing multiple drug-resistant tuberculosis to reveal fever, weight loss, and night sweats. Other symptoms of tuberculosis include fatigue and cough.

1. Crackles, cyanosis, and fever are symptoms of pneumonia.

3. Sudden chest pain, hemoptysis, and tachycardia are symptoms associated with pulmonary embolism.

4. Nausea, diaphoresis, and severe chest pain are consistent with an acute myocardial infarction.

Nursing Process: Assessing
Client Need: Physiological Integrity

10-43

③ Open chest wounds should be sealed (covered) with airtight dressings to prevent pneumothorax from developing or becoming worse.

1. The knife should be stabilized with a bulky dressing but not removed.

2. Cleansing the wound is not a priority.

4. The client should be placed in a semi-upright position, not supine.

Nursing Process: Implementing
Client Need: Safe, Effective Care Environment

1 0 - 4 4

③ **Initially, the nurse should assess the client for signs and symptoms of oxygen lack, document findings, and notify the physician.**

1. A drop in arterial oxygen pressure (P_2O_2) reflects changes in the client's oxygenation levels. Fifty mm Hg is below the normal range of 75 to 100 mm Hg and may indicate deterioration in the client's condition.

2. The physician will need to prescribe any changes in the type of oxygen delivery and its concentration; therefore, you would not increase the oxygen concentration until consultation with the physician.

4. After the initial assessment for signs and symptoms of oxygen lack, the nurse should continue to closely monitor the client's condition and report any changes to the physician.

Nursing Process: Evaluating
Client Need: Physiological Integrity

1 0 - 4 5

② **To evaluate the effectiveness of aminophylline, the nurse will monitor the rate and rhythm of the client's respirations. Aminophylline is a bronchodilator that relaxes the smooth muscle of the bronchi and relieves bronchospasm.**

1. Aminophylline does not affect the amount or color of secretions.

3. Aminophylline is not an antipyretic (agent that reduces fever).

4. Aminophylline does not expand the chest cavity. However, placing a client in an upright position will create more room for expansion of the diaphragm.

Nursing Process: Evaluating
Client Need: Physiological Integrity

1 0 - 4 6

③ **To provide safety during transport of a client with chest tubes, a pair of rubber-tipped forceps should be attached to the client's gown. It is important for the rubber-tipped forceps to be readily available should the chest tube become dislodged during the transport.**

1. The water-seal drainage should be kept upright and below chest level.

2. Chest tubes should never be clamped for prolonged periods of time, and, unless necessary, they should not be disconnected from the water-seal drainage.

4. Deep breaths will not prevent complications following chest tube dislodgment.

Nursing Process: Implementing
Client Need: Safe, Effective Care Environment

1 0 - 4 7

① The best method to use when administering oxygen to a client with amyotrophic lateral sclerosis is positive pressure ventilation. Positive pressure ventilation would ensure oxygen flow despite absence of spontaneous respirations. Clients in respiratory arrest cannot move air on their own. Supplemental oxygen would be indicated to combat hypoxemia. Amyotrophic lateral sclerosis is a syndrome characterized by muscular degeneration and atrophy.

2, 3, and 4. Clients who are not breathing on their own do not benefit from oxygen without ventilation.

Nursing Process: Planning
Client Need: Physiological Integrity

1 0 - 4 8

① **Administering analgesics and splinting with a pillow will provide the client who has a lung resection with the most comfort.**

2. Elevating the head of the bed will help the client to expectorate secretions from the lungs but it will not provide comfort.

3. Under most situations, chest tubes are not clamped. Clamped chest tubes may precipitate a tension pneumothorax.

4. Do not remove the client's oxygen. Coughing and deep breathing can deplete a client's oxygen reserve.

Nursing Process: Implementing
Client Need: Physiological Integrity

1 0 - 4 9

① **Clients receiving oxygen therapy by face mask should have their body temperature taken rectally. The flow of oxygen and humidity will affect the reading of an oral temperature.**

2. Receiving oxygen therapy by face mask will not interfere with a client's ability to participate in taking a bath.

3. Encouraging additional fluids is unnecessary since receiving oxygen by face mask does not dehydrate clients.

4. Receiving oxygen by face mask does not necessitate the need for coughing and deep breathing.

Nursing Process: Planning
Client Need: Physiological Integrity

10-50

③ **The nurse will place a client with chronic obstructive pulmonary disease (COPD) in an upright position to facilitate ventilation. An upright position of 90 degrees causes organs in the abdominal cavity to fall away from the diaphragm by gravity, thus giving the lungs more room to expand.**

1. Lying on the back with the face upward is referred to as supine (dorsal recumbent). This position is commonly used when examining a client's anterior chest and abdomen. It does not facilitate breathing.

2. A dorsal position with the head down and the feet elevated is contraindicated for clients experiencing respiratory distress because the abdominal organs press against the diaphragm and hinder breathing. This position may be used to treat clients in shock.

4. The left-side position is one in which the client is lying semi-prone on the left side with the right knee drawn up toward the chest. This position is commonly used when administering enemas. It does not facilitate breathing.

Nursing Process: Implementing
Client Need: Physiological Integrity

Practice Test 11

Mental Health Concepts, Communication, and Drug Abuse

11-1

For the past 6 weeks, you have administered chlorpromazine 50 mg tablets po qid to your client. Today, as you approach the client with her medication, she says she feels weak and that her mouth, gums, and throat are sore. You determine that she has a fever of 102°F. You will suspect:

1. acute dystonia.
2. early manifestations of agranulocytosis.
3. neuroleptic malignant syndrome.
4. xerostomia.

11-2

A client was admitted to the hospital complaining of abdominal pain and weight loss. The client is scheduled for diagnostic tests to rule out cancer. The client tells the nurse, "I am scared." Which statement by the nurse would be most appropriate?

1. "What diagnostic tests are you going to have?"
2. "Tell me what you're afraid of."
3. "There is nothing to be afraid of; we won't hurt you."
4. "If cancer is diagnosed early enough, there is a good chance of a cure."

11-3

You are communicating with a newly admitted client. Which communication technique can interfere with the establishment of a therapeutic relationship?

1. clarifying
2. summarizing
3. giving an opinion
4. providing information

1 1 - 4

You are caring for a group of people who were trapped for 2 hours inside the elevator of a burning building. Which of the following understandings will be especially useful in meeting the needs of these people?

1. Encouraging these individuals to tell and retell the experience will help reduce its psychological impact.
2. Allowing them to break into groups to discuss the experience will reinforce the psychological impact on each individual.
3. Permitting them to keep talking about the experience will result in an increase in self-pity.
4. Discouraging any discussion of the experience will help these people to handle their anxiety.

1 1 - 5

A client goes into a coma and death seems imminent. Which of the following measures would be most important for the nurse to implement at this time?

1. Maintain the client in a position of functional alignment.
2. Check the client's vital signs every 15 minutes.
3. Give the client skin and back care every hour.
4. Keep the client comfortable and the room quiet.

1 1 - 6

When caring for a client who has recently lost a body part or valued function, it is essential for the nurse to include which of the following measures in the care plan?

1. inviting the assistance of a person who has had a similar experience
2. encouraging an immediate independence in self-care
3. providing information to the client about how to contact community resources
4. allowing adequate time for the client to work through grief

11-7

A client has bulimia nervosa. During a binge, the client is most likely to consume:

1. fruits.
2. cakes and pies.
3. salads.
4. meats and breads.

11-8

Effective nursing management of clients who are dying requires the nurses caring for these clients to:

1. accept the inevitability of their own death.
2. recognize that loss and separation experiences are continual.
3. examine their own feelings and attitudes about dying.
4. understand that restoration of wellness is not possible.

11-9

A newly admitted client is unable to keep any schedule of activity due to an obsessive-compulsive hand-washing ritual. Which of the following nursing actions would be most appropriate for the client at this point in the hospitalization?

1. Waking the client early enough to perform the hand-washing rituals before scheduled activities begin.
2. Insisting that the client interrupt the rituals to attend scheduled activities.
3. Informing the client that ritualistic hand washing is interfering with scheduled activities.
4. Allowing the client to choose between completing the hand-washing rituals and going to the scheduled activities.

11-10

The mother of an 8-year-old calls the mental health clinic and tells the nurse, "My child has suddenly become intensely afraid of getting into the tub to take a bath. He is standing in the living room screaming uncontrollably. What should I do?" Which of the following information should the nurse give the mother?

1. "Hold your child snugly and speak in a soft voice to him."
2. "Have your child lie down and rest for a few minutes."
3. "Bring your child to the clinic as soon as possible."
4. "Tell your child that nothing is going to happen to him if he gets into the tub."

11-11

A daughter admits her mother into a nursing home after it was determined that her mother has organic brain syndrome. On a subsequent visit, the mother will not speak to the daughter. The daughter calls the nurse to ask if she should come the next day. Which of the following responses by the nurse would be best?

1. Advise the daughter to wait until her mother gives some indication that she is ready to see her.
2. Suggest that the daughter come back the next day since her continued interest will benefit the mother.
3. Tell the daughter that her mother will not miss her if she doesn't visit because she will become attached to staff members.
4. Tell the daughter that it is important for her mother to have visitors and suggest that she ask one of her friends to visit.

11-12

A client who was admitted to the medical-surgical unit with an acute gastrointestinal bleed is displaying a marked change in behavior. The client alternates between periods of talkativeness and stupor and frequently confabulates when talking. Because of the client's long history of alcohol abuse, you suspect:

1. Pick's disease.
2. Korsakoff-Wernicke syndrome.
3. Huntington's chorea.
4. epilepsy.

11-13

Which assessment finding is most likely to indicate child abuse?

1. parents who tell the nurse their 2-year-old seems ready for toilet training

2. parents who insist that their 2-year-old sit still for 30 minutes

3. an 18-month-old child with bruised areas on the forehead or knees

4. bluish-black areas on the buttocks of a newborn

11-14

The mother of a 6-year-old tells her child to put on his overshoes before going out into the rain. The child says, "No, they're too hard to put on." The mother turns to the nurse with a frustrated expression on her face. Which response by the nurse would be the most appropriate?

1. Say to the mother, "Maybe the overshoes are too small for the child's shoes."

2. Sit beside the child and say, "It's raining. You start pulling your overshoes on and I will help you with the hard part."

3. Hand the child the overshoes and say in a matter-of-fact manner, "If you will put the first one on, I'll put the second one on for you."

4. Say to the child, kindly but firmly, "You are trying to test your mother's authority; put your overshoes on right now."

11-15

A client is experiencing alcohol withdrawal syndrome. The nurse should be alert for which of the following complications of this condition?

1. aphasia

2. hypotension

3. diarrhea

4. convulsions

11-16

Your client is hyperactive, euphoric, and demonstrates inappropriate impulsive behavior. Which nursing intervention will be most beneficial in channeling the client's hyperactivity?

1. Encourage projects that offer motor activity in moderation.
2. Suggest participation in competitive activities.
3. Set firm limits on unacceptable behaviors.
4. Help the client become aware of underlying anger.

11-17

A client's wife says to the nurse, "I'd do anything to help my husband stop drinking." The primary goal of the nurse's response should be to:

1. help the client's wife to clarify the problem as she sees it.
2. encourage the client's wife to join a support group such as Al Anon.
3. tell the client's wife that she has done all she could possibly do to help her husband.
4. help the client's wife understand that alcoholism is a problem that only her husband can solve.

11-18

Because of chemotherapy, a client has lost all of his hair. The client appears distraught about his appearance and does not want to see anybody who comes to visit him. An appropriate nursing diagnosis for the client at this time is:

1. "dysfunctional grieving related to hair loss."
2. "defensive coping related to fear of rejection."
3. "body image disturbance related to body changes."
4. "impaired adjustment related to perceived threat."

11-19

A 2-year-old child has been hospitalized. The child's mother becomes upset when she comes to visit and the child turns his head away from her and holds his arms out to the nurse. The nurse will recognize that the most probable explanation for the child's behavior is:

1. he is angry with his mother for leaving him at the hospital.
2. he is testing the relationship between his mother and the nurse.
3. he now has a stronger emotional tie with the nurse than with his mother.
4. he is consciously trying to make his mother jealous.

11-20

A newborn is brought to the mother for the first time to be fed. The mother says to the nurse, "He's so little! I'm afraid I'll hurt him." Which of the following responses by the nurse would help to lessen the mother's fears?

1. "You can practice taking care of him while I am here."
2. "Is there someone at home who can help you care for him during the first few weeks?"
3. "You can watch me take care of the baby."
4. "The public health nurse can show you how to care for the baby when you get home."

11-21

Your client lost his job on New Year's Day. Since that time, he has lost weight, cries frequently, and is unable to sleep. He says he is "worthless." The nurse will associate the information obtained in the assessment with which of the following conditions?

1. dysthymia
2. seasonal affective disorder
3. bipolar disorder, depression
4. major depression, single episode

11-22

Which one of the following medications will the nurse associate with the treatment of impulsive drinking?

1. naltrexone
2. disulfiram
3. chlordiazepoxide
4. fluphenazine

11-23

As you walk into your client's room, you notice the client is crying and seems to be distraught. An appropriate response to the client's behavior would be to say:

1. "I'm so sorry to have invaded your privacy. I will come back later."
2. "You look upset; would you like to talk about it?"
3. "I'm sorry you're upset; let me get a tissue for you."
4. "You seem distraught; have you received bad news?"

11-24

Your client is experiencing acute mania. The client is easily distracted, disorganized, and extremely restless. Which of the following nursing actions will be most helpful in meeting the nutritional needs of this client?

1. Tell the client, "You may become sick if you do not eat."
2. Provide high-caloric foods the client can hold in the hand while moving about.
3. Place the client in a quiet environment with a tray of favorite foods.
4. Tell the client, "Unless you eat, you will have to receive tube feedings."

11-25

A client who has recently recovered from alcohol withdrawal syndrome tells the nurse, "I know I'm not perfect, but I'm not an alcoholic." This nurse will recognize the client's comment as an example of:

1. projection.
2. rationalization.
3. repression.
4. denial.

11-26

A client was brought to the Emergency Department following a heroin overdose. The nurse's first intervention will be to:

1. administer a narcotic antagonist.
2. apply a hypothermia blanket.
3. establish a patent airway.
4. prepare to aspirate gastric contents.

1 1 - 2 7

It has become necessary to use physical restraints on an aggressive client. To ensure the client's comfort, the nurse will check the restraints every:

1. 15 minutes.
2. 30 minutes.
3. 45 minutes.
4. hour.

1 1 - 2 8

A client experiencing severe depression was hospitalized following a suicide attempt. The client has been scheduled for electroconvulsive therapy. Immediately before the treatment, the client will receive the neuromuscular blocking agent:

1. Atropair.
2. Pentothal.
3. Anectine.
4. Brevital.

1 1 - 2 9

A client with Alzheimer's disease is confused and disoriented. The client frequently asks the nurse, "Will you help me find my room? I must have taken a wrong turn." Which comment by the nurse would be most therapeutic?

1. "You lead the way and I'll be here to help if you make a wrong turn."
2. "Come with me, I'll take you to your room."
3. "Your room is the first one on the right past the dining room."
4. "It's time for your exercise. Come with me to the recreational room."

1 1 - 3 0

Your client is receiving lithium to treat a bipolar affective disorder. Blood samples will be drawn to monitor the client's serum lithium levels. The nurse understands that the therapeutic maintenance level of lithium ranges from:

1. 0.2 to 0.9 mEq/L.
2. 0.4 to 1.0 mEq/L.
3. 1.6 to 2.4 mEq/L.
4. 2.2 to 3.2 mEq/L.

11-31

A client is hospitalized with ulcerative colitis and scheduled for an ileostomy. Prior to surgery, the nurse is reinforcing the need to cough and deep breathe. The client says, "Don't treat me like a child. I know how to breathe." Which of the following responses would be the most appropriate for the nurse to make?

1. "Do you know the reason for doing this?"
2. "Do you feel I'm talking down to you?"
3. "You're overreacting."
4. "No one else has had that complaint."

11-32

You are changing your client's ileostomy bag. It is most important to take which of the following measures?

1. Refrain from showing distaste.
2. Maintain strict surgical asepsis.
3. Explain the details of the procedure.
4. Wipe the stoma with a mild antiseptic.

11-33

Your client is experiencing the manic phase of a bipolar disorder. The client is unkempt, profane, and hyperactive. Which nursing intervention would be the most therapeutic when the client's language becomes profane and abusive?

1. Let the client know the language being used is unacceptable.
2. Isolate the client from others until profane and abusive language is discontinued.
3. Ignore the client's attempts to get attention by using profane and abusive language.
4. Recognize the client's language as a part of the illness and set firm limits.

11-34

Your client is having delusions of persecution and refuses to eat. The client says the personnel are poisoning the food. Which one of the following responses by the nurse would be most appropriate initially in coping with this situation?

1. Permit the client to eat food that has been brought from home.
2. Tell the client, "No one is putting poison in your food."
3. Taste the client's food and say, "See, I told you there was no poison in your food."
4. Recognize the client's behavior as a symptom of the condition.

11-35

Your client has bulimia nervosa. Maintenance of desired body weight is achieved by clients with bulimia by:

1. consuming a less-than-adequate amount of an otherwise well-balanced diet.
2. restricting high-caloric foods during binges.
3. premeditated binges.
4. self-induced vomiting along with laxative and diuretic abuse.

11-36

Your client is experiencing delusions of persecution. You are to administer the client's antipsychotic medication for the first time. Which one of the following actions would be most likely to ensure the client's acceptance of the medication?

1. Administer the medication when the client does not appear to be upset or delusional.
2. Request additional standby personnel in the event the client refuses to take the medication.
3. Explain the procedure for administering the medication prior to approaching the client.
4. Attempt to disguise the client's medication in food and drink.

11-37

Which one of the following nursing actions would be most effective in preventing a client who is a suicidal risk from committing suicide?

1. administering antidepressant medication
2. knowing the whereabouts of the client at all times
3. providing opportunities for the client to express thoughts and feelings
4. encouraging participation in ward activities

11-38

A client who is going to be discharged tells the nurse, "I'm afraid I won't be able to pay all my medical bills." Which comment by the nurse would facilitate further elaboration by the client?

1. "I'll introduce you to the social workers. They will be able to help you."
2. "I'll report your concern to the business office."
3. "I understand how you feel. The cost of health care is alarming."
4. "You seem worried about this situation."

11-39

A plan of care for an infant with fetal alcohol syndrome should place the most emphasis on overcoming problems involving:

1. fluid balance.
2. peripheral circulation.
3. nutrition.
4. airway clearance.

11-40

Your client has been diagnosed with hypochondriasis following a complete physical examination. The client was informed that no organic basis for the presenting complaints was found. The client tells you, "I'm sure I have a terrible disease." Your best response would be to:

1. ignore the client's complaints.
2. reaffirm the medical findings.
3. ask the client, "Why do you think you are ill?"
4. tell the client she looks healthy.

11-41

A client was hospitalized following a suicide attempt after losing a job. One week later, you observe a sudden apparent improvement in the client. The nurse understands that the most probable reason for the apparent improvement is that the client:

1. has gotten some information about a new job.
2. has established supportive relationships with the personnel.
3. has been relieved of a stressful work environment.
4. may be committed to suicide and has a workable plan.

11-42

While watching the evening news on the television, a delusional client shouts, "You can't blame me for dropping that bomb." The nurse will recognize the client's behavior as a response to:

1. an hallucination.
2. an idea of reference.
3. an illusion.
4. a delusion of persecution.

11-43

You are planning activities for a client who has an obsessive-compulsive disorder. You will choose times for the activities when the client is relatively anxiety-free. You understand the client's anxiety will be at its lowest:

1. immediately following the performance of the ritualistic behavior.
2. during the time the ritualistic behavior is being performed.
3. nearing the completion of the ritualistic behavior.
4. immediately before the performance of the ritualistic behavior.

11-44

A client with terminal cancer tells the nurse, "I'm dying." The most therapeutic response by the nurse would be:

1. "It must be frightening to know that you are dying."
2. "Tell me more about how you feel."
3. "There is always hope that a treatment will be available that might save your life."
4. "You really look much better."

11-45

An 8-year-old client has hemophilia. Which statement by the client would reflect the child's acceptance of the constant seriousness of the condition?

1. "I use a Water Pik for cleaning my teeth."
2. "I take Tylenol if I have pain."
3. "I wear a Medic-alert identification bracelet."
4. "I keep an emergency kit at my bedside."

11-46

A client is receiving haloperidol 5 mg po tid. To protect the client from a frequent side effect of this medication, the nurse will:

1. provide the client with a low-sodium diet.
2. instruct the client to rise slowly to a standing position.
3. restrict fluid intake to 1000 cc daily.
4. provide a diet that is free of cheese products.

11-47

Prior to admission to the hospital, a 2-year-old child was partially bowel trained but now defecates involuntarily. The nurse's approach to this situation should be based on which of the following assessments?

1. What is the child's reaction to the soiling?
2. How compulsive is the child about cleanliness?
3. Is the child too young for bowel training?
4. Is bowel training important to the child?

11-48

A 45-year-old client is admitted to an alcoholic treatment center. He has been drinking a quart or more of liquor a day for 10 to 15 years. The client has been drinking up to the time of admission. In responding to long-term alcohol abuse, the nurse admitting the client would expect the immediate treatment to include which of the following prescriptions?

1. oral fluids and a narcotic
2. a cool bath, a barbiturate, and blood lithium levels
3. regular diet as tolerated, thiamine, and a tranquilizer
4. a spinal tap, bromides, and restraints

11-49

Your client has just awakened from an electroconvulsive therapy treatment. The most appropriate nursing action at this time would be to:

1. arrange for the client's diet to be served.
2. orient the client.
3. observe the client for signs of suicidal behavior.
4. provide the client with a quiet environment in which to rest.

11-50

A mother asks the nurse, "What are those little white spots all over my baby's face? None of my other babies had them." Which of the following responses would be best?

1. "They are called milia and will soon disappear."
2. "Most babies have them; there is no need to worry."
3. "You should not be concerned about such small cysts."
4. "Some babies have many more spots than your baby."

Practice Test 11

Answers, Rationales, and Explanations

1 1 - 1

② **The nurse will suspect the early development of agranulocytosis (an acute disease characterized by a deficit or total lack of granulocytic white blood cells), a rare occurrence that is potentially fatal. Chlorpromazine (Thorazine) would be discontinued and reverse isolation instituted along with stat blood work.**

1. Dystonia is characterized by painful spasms of voluntary muscles affecting the neck, back, jaws, limbs, and eyes. Dystonia is usually seen in the first 5 days of neuroleptic administration.

3. Neuroleptic malignant syndrome (NMS) is a rare, idiosyncratic reaction to neuroleptic agents characterized by muscle rigidity, hyperthermia, and stupor. There is an increase in white blood cells.

4. Xerostomia is dryness of the mouth caused by reduction in the amount of saliva. Xerostomia is a common side effect associated with the administration of neuroleptic medications like Thorazine.

Nursing Process: Analyzing

Client Need: Psychosocial Integrity

1 1 - 2

② **The nurse's best response would include an open-ended statement such as, "Tell me what you're afraid of." This allows the client an opportunity to verbalize fears.**

1. The client is not afraid of the diagnostic tests. The client is afraid the tests will indicate the presence of cancer.

3. Telling the client there is nothing to be afraid of is not realistic. It is the possible test results that are causing the fear.

4. Suggesting that early detection of cancer will give the client a "good chance" also suggests that if the cancer is advanced, the client won't have a "good chance."

Nursing Process: Implementing

Client Need: Psychosocial Integrity

1 1 - 3

③ **Giving an opinion can be detrimental when a nurse is trying to build a relationship with a client. Giving an opinion takes decision making away from the client. It inhibits spontaneity, stalls problem solving, and creates doubt. Giving an opinion prevents the client from developing solutions.**

1, 2, and 4. Therapeutic techniques of communication include clarifying, summarizing, and providing information. These techniques help to build a relationship.

Nursing Process: Implementing

Client Need: Psychosocial Integrity

11-4

① **Repeated telling of a harrowing experience allows the people involved to reflect, recognize the importance of the experience in their lives, and begin the process of mastering the experience.**

2. Perpetuating a discussion of the experience should be done to reduce its impact, not to reinforce the impact.

3. Self-pity should not be a goal but one of a series of stages that may be experienced by some individuals who have had a harrowing experience.

4. Avoiding the discussion of a terrifying experience prevents individuals from working through the trauma and coping effectively.

Nursing Process: Implementing
Client Need: Psychosocial Integrity

11-5

④ **When the death of a client appears imminent, nursing measures should focus on the client's comfort and the preservation of a quiet environment.**

1. Following the death of a client, the nurse should maintain the client's body in a position of functional alignment. This will assist in the preparation of the body for burial.

2 and 3. Taking the client's vital signs or giving back care serves no purpose under the circumstances.

Nursing Process: Implementing
Client Need: Psychosocial Integrity

11-6

④ **When caring for a client who has lost a body part or valued function, the nursing care plan should include measures that allow adequate time for the client to work through the grief. Any loss, real or perceived, requires a period of time for grieving. Mourning is a well-defined psychological process by which grief is resolved. Encouraging the client's expression of feelings and listening are most important in caring for the grieving client.**

1. Inviting the assistance of a person who has had a similar loss can be helpful once the client has worked through the grieving process.

2. Encouraging immediate independence and self-care may overwhelm the client.

3. Providing information about community resources should be done when the client has worked through the grieving process and is psychologically ready.

Nursing Process: Planning
Client Need: Psychosocial Integrity

1 1 - 7

② **When binging, clients with bulimia nervosa will select high-caloric foods, such as cakes and pies, which require little chewing and are easily ingested. Bulimia is characterized by excessive food intake accompanied by purging.**

1. Fruits may be ingested during the phase of food restrictions, but during a binge, fruits would not be selected because they are not typically high-caloric or as easily ingested as cakes and pies.

3. Salads are not foods of choice during a binge. However, during the restrictive phase, these clients would likely select salads due to their low-caloric value.

4. Meats and breads are not easily ingested and therefore are not selected during a binge. These foods also require more chewing than items such as cakes and pies.

Nursing Process: Assessing

Client Need: Psychosocial Integrity

1 1 - 8

③ **To effectively care for dying clients, nurses must first examine their own feelings and attitudes about dying.**

1. Effective nursing care of dying clients requires more than an academic or intellectual acceptance of death.

2. Just recognizing that loss and separation are continual would not help nurses to care for dying clients and their unique needs as they approach death.

4. Understanding that wellness is not possible for the dying client is helpful to the extent that the nurse will be less likely to deny the needs of those clients. However, examining one's own feelings about dying is essential when caring for those who are dying.

Nursing Process: Planning

Client Need: Psychosocial Integrity

11-9

① **Waking the client early enough to complete the hand-washing ritual and still have time to attend scheduled meetings will help to involve the client in the milieu. Early on in the client's hospitalization, it would be important for the client to understand that no one is going to try to prevent the ritualistic hand washing.**

2. The purpose of obsessive-compulsive behavior is to relieve anxiety. Interrupting the rituals will only increase the client's anxiety.

3. Informing the client that the hand-washing ritual is interfering with scheduled activities will not only increase anxiety but it will place the client in a dilemma.

4. The client should not be placed in a position to choose between performing a hand-washing ritual and going to scheduled activities.

Nursing Process: Implementing

Client Need: Psychosocial Integrity

11-10

① **The mother should be told to hold her child snugly and speak softly to him. The child is demonstrating behavior suggestive of a phobia. He is unable to control his anxiety and fears and needs someone to take control of him and the situation.**

2. A child who is out of control because of fear and anxiety is unable to lie down and rest.

3. Bringing the child to the clinic before helping him to gain control will only prolong the fear and anxiety he is experiencing.

4. Attempting to reason with a person who has a phobia is inappropriate since a phobia is an irrational fear.

Nursing Process: Implementing

Client Need: Psychosocial Integrity

11-11

② **The nurse should suggest that the daughter come back to see her mother since the daughter's continued interest will benefit her mother. Consistent family contact is important in providing stability in the environment of a client with organic brain syndrome. Socializing can improve the client's quality of life.**

1. Clients with organic brain syndrome (pathological dysfunction of the brain) are not likely to initiate visits. It will be up to the client's daughter to plan and implement visits with the client.

3. The daughter's visit will be beneficial for her mother. The nurse should encourage socialization with family members.

4. Advising the daughter conveys that the nurse knows best and that the daughter cannot think for herself. This approach fosters dependency and hinders problem solving.

Nursing Process: Implementing

Client Need: Psychosocial Integrity

11-12

② **The nurse will suspect Korsakoff-Wernicke syndrome. Korsakoff-Wernicke syndrome, which involves disorientation, delirium, and inappropriate phrasing, is associated with long-term alcohol abuse.**

1. Pick's disease (Alzheimer's disease) is a form of presenile dementia due to atrophy of the frontal and temporal lobes of the brain. The etiology is unknown.

3. Huntington's chorea is an inherited disease that is typified by involuntary face and limb movements.

4. Seizure activity is the hallmark of epilepsy.

Nursing Process: Evaluating
Client Need: Physiological Integrity

11-13

② **Parents who insist that their 2-year-old sit still for 30 minutes may attempt to enforce their demands in abusive ways. It is unrealistic for the parents of a 2-year-old to expect the child to sit still for 30 minutes.**

1. It is appropriate for parents of a 2-year-old to expect the child to be ready for toilet training. A child cannot voluntarily control bowel and bladder sphincters until myelinization of the spinal cord occurs. Myelinization takes place between 12 and 18 months of age.

3. It would be appropriate for an 18-month-old to have bruised areas on the forehead and knees. At this age, children are often falling in their attempts to walk.

4. Mongolian spots (bluish-black areas on the buttocks and thighs of a newborn) are normally seen in 80% of nonwhite newborns and 10% of white newborns. The spots fade away with age.

Nursing Process: Assessing
Client Need: Psychosocial Integrity

11-14

② The nurse should let the child know that help will be given with the "hard part" of putting on shoes. Children 6 years of age, like all children, need to have set limits. Compliance can be facilitated by giving the child an explanation for why the overshoes are needed. Also, limits are set and the child is not left without help if needed.

1. Suggesting that the overshoes may be too tight ignores the child's attempt to challenge his mother's authority.

3. Bargaining with the child puts the child in control and does not set limits on his behavior. If the child refuses to keep his end of the bargain, the situation is likely to escalate.

4. Even though the child is testing his mother's authority, it is not necessary for the nurse to verbalize the psychodynamics of the interaction. Challenging the child with a demand could escalate the situation unnecessarily.

Nursing Process: Implementing

Client Need: Psychosocial Integrity

11-15

④ The nurse should be alert for convulsions when clients are withdrawing from alcohol. Alcohol lowers the seizure threshold in vulnerable individuals. The sudden absence of alcohol from the system of an alcoholic may precipitate convulsions.

1. Aphasia is the absence or impairment of the ability to communicate by speaking, writing, or use of signs. It is due to dysfunction of the brain centers. Aphasia is a clinical manifestation of cerebrovascular accidents.

2. Clients who experience alcohol withdrawal are likely to have hypertension and tachycardia.

3. Nausea and vomiting may be experienced by clients in alcohol withdrawal. However, diarrhea is not a typical symptom.

Nursing Process: Assessing

Client Need: Physiological Integrity

11-16

① Encouraging projects that offer motor activity in moderation can help diffuse hyperactivity.

2. Competitive activities are harmful because they further stimulate the hyperactive client.

3. Setting firm limits is essential but does not defuse hyperactivity.

4. The attention span of the hyperactive client is extremely short and does not allow for interventions that focus on gaining insight.

Nursing Process: Implementing

Client Need: Safe, Effective Care Environment

11-17

① **The nurse's primary goal will be to help the client's wife clarify the problem as she sees it. This will help the nurse to know how to proceed.**

2. Suggesting a support group such as Al Anon would be inappropriate before determining how the wife of the client views the problem.

3. Telling the client's wife that she has done all she could possibly do to help her husband is avoiding the wife's concern by attempting to placate her.

4. Alcoholics can be helped by others but it's important for those who want to help to know how to help.

Nursing Process: Planning

Client Need: Psychosocial Integrity

11-18

③ **An appropriate nursing diagnosis at this time would be, "Body image disturbance related to body changes." This diagnosis is evidenced by verbal and nonverbal responses to actual or perceived changes in the structure and function of the client's body.**

1. Grieving is an expression of distress at loss and is generally considered to be dysfunctional when it is prolonged or sustained (usually a year after the loss).

2. "Defensive coping related to fear of rejection" includes denial of problems, projection of blame onto others, and an attitude of superiority toward others.

4. "Impaired adjustment related to the perceived threat" includes the inability to modify lifestyle to accommodate change.

Nursing Process: Analyzing

Client Need: Psychosocial Integrity

11-19

① **The nurse will recognize that the most likely explanation for the child's behavior is anger toward his mother for leaving him at the hospital. The client is unable to understand why his mother left. A 2-year-old child has a strong attachment to his mother and needs to be close to her. Loss of contact will result in behavior that is manifested as fear and anger.**

2. Testing relationships between adults will develop when the child is older. Children will test the relationship between their parents by pitting one parent against the other in an attempt to get their way about something such as the purchase of a new toy.

3. The child does not have a stronger bond with the nurse. The child is demonstrating his anger and fear by rejecting his mother at the moment.

4. A 2-year-old does not understand the abstract concept of jealousy.

Nursing Process: Analyzing

Client Need: Psychosocial Integrity

11-20

1. **Assuring the new mother that she can practice caring for her baby while under supervision may decrease her anxiety. The nurse's comment indicates her confidence in the new mother's ability to care for her baby.**

2. Asking the new mother if someone at home can help her take care of her baby for a few weeks is inappropriate. The nurse should recognize the mother's concern and proceed to assess the client's strengths and weaknesses for caring for her baby.

3. Telling the new mother that she can learn how to take care of her baby by watching the nurse take care of the baby is placing the mother in a passive observer role. The mother should have the opportunity to actually participate in her baby's care while under supervision.

4. The client can be taught how to take care of her baby now. The nurse can teach her a great deal about taking care of her baby before she leaves the hospital. Waiting for a public health nurse to teach the mother is ignoring the mother's present need.

Nursing Process: Implementing
Client Need: Psychosocial Integrity

11-21

4. **The nurse will associate the information obtained during assessment with a major depression, single episode. There is evidence to suggest a great change from the client's previous functions. The client is unable to function socially or occupationally. The client is experiencing insomnia, weight loss, and is in constant emotional discomfort.**

1. Dysthymia occurs over a 2-year period and is considered mild to moderate in degree. Clients with dysthymia are at risk for developing major depressive conditions. Clients with dysthymia experience anadonia (inability to find pleasure in anything).

2. Seasonal affective disorder (SAD) is characterized by hypersomnia, fatigue, weight gain, irritability, and difficulties with interpersonal relationships. This condition usually occurs in the winter and is effectively treated with 2 to 3 hours of bright light daily.

3. Bipolar disorders are mood disorders that include one or more manic episodes and one or more depressive episodes.

Nursing Process: Assessing
Client Need: Psychosocial Integrity

11-22

② The nurse will associate disulfiram (Antabuse) with the treatment of impulsive drinking. It is usually given to alcoholics who have demonstrated the ability to stay sober. Clients drinking alcohol while taking this drug will experience the alcohol-disulfiram reaction. Symptoms of this reaction include facial flushing, nausea, vomiting, hypertension, respiratory distress and profuse sweating.

1. The medication naltrexone (ReVia) is an agent used to treat alcoholics by decreasing the client's craving for alcohol. This medication is not given to treat impulsive drinking.

3. Chlordiazepoxide (Librium) is administered to treat the symptoms of alcohol withdrawal, not impulsive drinking.

4. Fluphenazine (Prolixin) is an antipsychotic that is administered to treat acute and chronic psychoses. There is no association with this drug and the treatment of alcoholism.

Nursing Process: Implementing
Client Need: Psychosocial Integrity

11-23

② It would be appropriate for the nurse to say, "You look upset; would you like to talk about it?" This response acknowledges that the client is upset and provides the client with an opportunity to express feelings.

1. Leaving the room of a client who is crying and upset is inappropriate. The nurse who would do this is probably feeling incapable of relieving the client's emotional pain and is using the client's need for privacy as an excuse to leave.

3. Suggesting that you get a tissue for a client who is upset and crying is focusing on the physical aspects of the situation (runny nose and tears). It would be more therapeutic to focus on the underlying cause of the crying.

4. Instead of trying to guess what has upset the client, the nurse should acknowledge that the client seems upset and provide the client with an opportunity to talk about the problem.

Nursing Process: Assessing
Client Need: Psychosocial Integrity

11-24

② The nurse will provide hyperactive clients with high-caloric foods that can be held in the hand and eaten as the client moves about. Examples of high-caloric "finger-foods" include milk shakes and pastries. Constipation is also a concern; therefore, fiber and fluids are encouraged by providing fruits that can be eaten while the client is moving about.

1 and 4. It is not possible to reason with clients who are experiencing acute mania. They have a short attention span and are unable to concentrate.

3. Clients who are experiencing acute mania are unable to sit still. Placing them in a quiet, non-stimulating environment with favorite foods will not solve the problem.

Nursing Process: Planning

Client Need: Physiological Integrity

11-25

④ The nurse will recognize that the client is using the defense mechanism (DM) of denial. Defense mechanisms are unconscious, intrapsychic processes used by clients to ward off feelings of anxiety by preventing conscious awareness of threatening feelings. By using denial, the client is escaping the unpleasant realities of what it means to be an alcoholic.

1. Projection occurs when one attributes one's own intolerable attributes to another person, such as an alcoholic who accuses someone else of being an alcoholic.

2. Rationalization occurs when one attempts to present acceptable explanations for an intolerable attribute. An alcoholic might say, "If you had the job I have, you would drink, too."

Nursing Process: Assessing

Client Need: Psychosocial Integrity

11-26

③ The nurse's first intervention when caring for a client who has had a heroin overdose is to establish a patent airway. Heroin overdose requires immediate intervention to prevent death.

1. Following the establishment of a patent airway, the nurse would administer the narcotic antagonist naloxone (Narcan). This medication quickly reverses central nervous system depression.

2. A hypothermia blanket would be appropriate for a client who had taken an overdose of a stimulant, such as cocaine.

4. Aspirating gastric contents would be necessary when caring for a client who had taken an overdose of a sedative/hypnotic.

Nursing Process: Planning

Client Need: Physiological Integrity

11-27

(1) **If it becomes necessary to physically restrain a client, the nurse will know to check the restraints every 15 minutes. Frequent position changes, massaging the skin, and range-of-motion exercises are all helpful in preventing prolonged pressure against blood vessels and nerves.**

2, 3, and 4. Waiting longer than 15 minutes to assess a client in restraints could place a client in jeopardy. The goal of restraints is safety for the client and others.

Nursing Process: Implementing
Client Need: Psychosocial Integrity

11-28

(3) **Immediately before an electroconvulsive therapy treatment, the nurse will administer the neuromuscular blocking agent succinylcholine (Anectine). Anectine is a neuromuscular blocking agent (muscle relaxant) that is used after induction of anesthesia to promote muscle paralysis. When administered intravenously immediately prior to electroconvulsive therapy (ECT), it relaxes muscles and prevents the risk of fractures and soft tissue injuries.**

1. Approximately 30 to 60 minutes before electroconvulsive therapy, the nurse will administer atropine (Atropair) intramuscularly. Atropine is an anticholinergic that will decrease oral and respiratory secretions.

2 and 4. Methohexital sodium (Brevital) and thiopental (Pentothal) are both short-acting anesthetics, either of which may be given just prior to the neuromuscular blocking agent Anectine.

Nursing Process: Implementing
Client Need: Psychosocial Integrity

11-29

(2) **The nurse should say, "Come with me, I'll take you to your room." Clients with Alzheimer's disease have progressive, irreversible memory loss and deterioration of intellect. They experience confusion and disorientation.**

1. The client is confused and disoriented and unable to lead the way. Asking the client to lead the way is setting the client up for failure.

3. The client is unable to follow directions due to short-term memory loss, confusion, and disorientation.

4. Diverting the client's attention is avoiding the client's immediate need for orientation.

Nursing Process: Implementing
Client Need: Psychosocial Integrity

11-30

②   **The nurse knows that the therapeutic maintenance level of lithium (Lithotabs) ranges from 0.4 to 1.0 mEq/L. To prevent toxicity, lithium maintenance levels should not exceed 1.5 mEq/L.**

1.   In order to be therapeutic, lithium levels should fall between 0.4 and 1.0 mEq/L. A lithium level below 0.4 would not be therapeutic.

3.   A lithium level between 1.6 and 2.4 could cause signs of advanced to severe lithium toxicity such as mental confusion, uncoordination, ataxia, stupor, and death.

4.   A lithium level between 2.2 and 3.2 mEq/L could cause severe toxicity and death. Hemodialysis may be considered in such cases.

Nursing Process: Evaluating

Client Need: Psychosocial Integrity

11-31

②   **It would be appropriate for the nurse to respond with "Do you feel I'm talking down to you?" This response shows respect for the client's feelings and allows the client to calm down. The nurse should keep communications open despite the fact that the client is upset.**

1.   Asking the client "Do you know the reason for doing this?" may put the client on the defensive and is not recommended.

3.   Saying "You're overreacting" is minimizing the client's feelings and is judgmental.

4.   Saying "No one else has had that complaint" is suggesting that the client's response is somehow out of the ordinary and therefore should be ignored.

Nursing Process: Implementing

Client Need: Safe, Effective Care Environment

11-32

(1) **The nurse should not demonstrate an attitude of distaste when changing a client's ileostomy bag. The client is likely to have feelings of embarrassment and a body image disturbance. Most clients with ileostomies worry about odor control and bowel excretion. They will take the attitude of the nurse as an example of the way other people will react. By not showing distaste when changing the client's ileostomy bag, the nurse is teaching the client not to be embarrassed about caring for the ileostomy.**

2. There is no need to use sterile technique when changing a client's ileostomy bag. The gastrointestinal tract is not sterile.

3. There is no indication that the nurse is teaching the client how to change the ileostomy bag, only that the bag is being changed.

4. The stoma should be cleansed with gentle friction using mild soap and warm water. The skin should be patted dry. An antiseptic would be irritating to the skin.

Nursing Process: Implementing

Client Need: Psychosocial Integrity

11-33

(4) **The nurse will recognize the client's language as part of the illness and set firm limits. The client's offensive language is an outlet for uncomfortable, hyperactive feelings that the client is unable to control.**

1. The client is not able to control the illness responsible for the profane and abusive language. Therefore, telling the client that the language is unacceptable is inappropriate.

2. The nurse should help the client to redirect the hyperactivity that underlies the use of profane and abusive language.

3. A manic client who is out of control should not be ignored. The nurse should provide structure and set limits that will help the client feel secure. Hyperactive clients want to know that someone is in control.

Nursing Process: Implementing

Client Need: Psychosocial Integrity

11-34

④ **The nurse should recognize the client's delusion as a symptom of the condition.**

1. Permitting the client to eat food that was brought from home is not therapeutic because it implies that the food served in the hospital is poisoned.

2. Delusions are false, fixed ideas or beliefs. Simply telling a client that no one is poisoning the food will be totally ineffective.

3. A client who saw the nurse taste the food would not be convinced that the food wasn't poisoned. The client would reason that the nurse had tasted the part of the food that did not have poison in it.

Nursing Process: Implementing

Client Need: Psychosocial Integrity

11-35

④ **Clients with bulimia nervosa attempt to maintain their body weight by self-induced vomiting (purging), laxative and diuretic abuse, exercise, and avoidance of food (fasting) in between bouts of binging.**

1. Clients with bulimia do not eat a well-balanced diet. They have a pattern of fasting and then consuming large quantities of less-than-healthy foods.

2. During binges, these clients consume extremely large quantities of high-caloric, easily ingested foods such as milk shakes, cakes, and pies.

3. Binges are not always preplanned. In fact, binges may be associated with problems of impulse control.

Nursing Process: Assessing

Client Need: Psychosocial Integrity

11-36

③ **To facilitate compliance, the nurse should explain the procedure for administering medications. An explanation may help to establish a therapeutic rapport based on mutual respect and trust.**

1. The nurse should not assume that because a client does not appear to be upset or delusional that the client is rational and calm.

2. Requesting additional standby personnel is likely to be interpreted by a suspicious, delusional client as a threat.

4. Any attempt to deceive the client will compromise credibility and is inappropriate.

Nursing Process: Implementing

Client Need: Psychosocial Integrity

11-37

② **Knowing the whereabouts of clients who are suicidal should be the nurse's first consideration. It is an established fact that clients who have committed suicide have done so in very short periods of time. The nurse who knows the location of clients at all times can be assured of the their physical safety.**

1. Whereas the administration of medication should not be minimized, the nurse should not think that clients who are at risk would not take their own lives simply because they are receiving medication. The fact that clients may need to take medications can be a contributing factor in their decision to attempt suicide.

3. Providing opportunities for suicidal clients to express their thoughts and feelings outwardly, as opposed to turning their anger inward, is therapeutic. However, it may not be sufficient in deterring clients from taking their own lives.

4. Participation in ward activities gives clients who are at risk an opportunity to concentrate on something other than planning suicide. Physical activities can also be helpful in channeling potentially destructive behaviors. However, activities alone do not solve the underlying problems that contribute to the choice some clients make to take their lives.

Nursing Process: Implementing

Client Need: Psychosocial Integrity

11-38

④ **The nurse could facilitate further elaboration from the client by saying, "You seem worried about this situation." By identifying the client's feelings, the nurse opens the conversation for additional comments by the client.**

1 and 2. Telling the client that you will contact the business office or a social worker will bring the conversation to an abrupt end. The client will be left to worry about a problem that was not fully expressed.

3. Agreeing with clients doesn't leave them with an option to change their point of view or their feelings.

Nursing Process: Implementing

Client Need: Psychosocial Integrity

11-39

③ **Poor feeding is usually a problem for infants with fetal alcohol syndrome during infancy. Feeding difficulties are related to a poor suck reflex, microcephaly, irritability, and later hyperactivity. Other characteristics of infants with fetal alcohol syndrome are hypotonia, mental retardation, motor retardation, hearing disorders, and growth retardation as well as facial features that include thin upper lip, hypoplastic maxilla, and short, upturned nose.**

1, 2, and 4. Fluid balance, peripheral circulation, and airway clearance are not problems typically associated with fetal alcohol syndrome.

Nursing Process: Planning
Client Need: Psychosocial Integrity

11-40

② **The nurse should reaffirm the medical findings. Consistently reaffirming the medical findings is the most appropriate response to give clients who are experiencing hypochondriasis. This will expose the client to the facts.**

1. Ignoring the client would convey a lack of interest and would be inappropriate.

3. Asking the client "Why do you think you are ill?" will give the client an audience for verbalizing complaints.

4. Telling the client "You look healthy" will provide an opportunity for the client to go through a list of complaints.

Nursing Process: Implementing
Client Need: Psychosocial Integrity

11-41

④ **The most probable reason for sudden apparent improvement in a suicidal client is that the client may be committed to suicide and has a workable plan. This sudden improvement comes about as a consequence of the client resolving all ambivalence about committing suicide.**

1. There is no indication that the client has received any information about a new job.

2. There would be a gradual improvement in a client who developed supportive, therapeutic relationships with the personnel, not a sudden, overall improvement.

3. Occasionally a client will show improvement when hospitalized and relieved of a stressful environment. However, when this happens, the improvement is usually immediate, not a week after hospitalization.

Nursing Process: Assessing
Client Need: Psychosocial Integrity

11-42

② **The nurse will recognize the client's behavior as a response to an idea of reference. Ideas of reference are false ideas (delusions) that outside occurrences have special meaning to oneself.**

1. An hallucination is a perception of the senses for which no external stimulus exists; for example, a person who hears people talking when no people are present.

3. An illusion is a misinterpretation of reality. For example, a client says there are bugs in an ashtray when in reality the ashtray is filled with cigarette butts.

4. A delusion of persecution is a false idea or belief that people are plotting against you. For example, a client says all of his coworkers are jealous of him and are trying to kill him.

Nursing Process: Assessing
Client Need: Psychosocial Integrity

11-43

① **Clients who have obsessive-compulsive disorders are the least anxious immediately after the ritualistic behavior has been completed.**

2 and 3. Interrupting an obsessive-compulsive client at any point during the performance of the ritualistic behavior will increase anxiety. Many clients feel they have to start the ritual all over again from the beginning once they are interrupted.

4. Clients are the most anxious immediately before the ritualistic behavior is performed.

Nursing Process: Planning
Client Need: Psychosocial Integrity

11-44

② **A client who is dying can benefit from a broad opening statement that encourages expression of feelings, such as, "Tell me more about how you feel."**

1. Suggesting to the client, "It must be frightening to know you are dying," is based on the assumption that the client is frightened. This may not be the case.

3. Telling dying clients that a life-saving treatment might be found that will save their lives is inappropriate and prevents clients from preparing for death.

4. Telling dying clients, "You really look much better," is a barrier to further therapeutic communication. It signals the nurse's unwillingness to converse with the client about impending death.

Nursing Process: Implementing
Client Need: Psychosocial Integrity

1 1 - 4 5

③ **Wearing a Medic-alert bracelet demonstrates a constant awareness of the seriousness of hemophilia. If clients with hemophilia are ever unconscious, it can still be determined that they have hemophilia.**

1. It is not necessary for clients with hemophilia to use a Water Pik. A soft bristle toothbrush softened in warm water is acceptable for mouth care.

2. Tylenol for pain is an appropriate choice. However, it is less important than wearing a Medic-alert bracelet.

4. Keeping an emergency kit at the bedside is not likely to be of much use. Accidents are not likely to occur in bed.

Nursing Process: Assessing

Client Need: Psychosocial Integrity

1 1 - 4 6

② **Clients receiving haloperidol (Haldol) should be advised to make position changes slowly to minimize the potential for orthostatic hypotension.**

1. A low-sodium diet may be prescribed for a client who is experiencing hypertension, not hypotension.

3. Fluids should be encouraged since clients have a tendency to become dehydrated.

4. Clients who are taking monoamine oxidase (MAO) inhibitors are to avoid foods with tyramine. Hypertensive crisis may occur with the ingestion of foods containing high amounts of tyramine. Foods containing tyramine include aged cheese, wine, pickled or smoked fish, overripe fruits, and foods containing Aspartame.

Nursing Process: Implementing

Client Need: Psychosocial Integrity

1 1 - 4 7

① **The nurse's approach to this problem should be based on the child's reaction to the soiling. It is normal to expect some degree of regression with hospitalization.**

2 and 4. Overreacting and overanalyzing the child's behavior is not beneficial or relevant.

3. A 2-year-old is physically mature enough to be bowel trained and had demonstrated progress in that direction before hospitalization.

Nursing Process: Assessing

Client Need: Psychosocial Integrity

1 1 - 4 8

③ **The nurse would anticipate a treatment plan that included a regular diet as tolerated, thiamine, and a tranquilizer. Nutritional deficiency is a major problem exhibited by individuals with a long history of alcohol abuse. Thiamine is used to retard peripheral neuropathy common in long-term alcohol abuse. A deficiency of thiamine may also lead to Korsakoff's syndrome. Tranquilizers may be used as a detoxification agent to prevent delirium tremens.**

1. Encouraging oral fluids is recommended since the client is likely to be dehydrated. However, narcotics are contraindicated because they are central nervous system (CNS) depressants and potentiate the depressant effects of alcohol.

2. The client is not receiving lithium (Lithotabs). There is no need to draw blood for lithium levels. Also, barbiturates are central nervous system (CNS) depressants and should not be taken because they potentiate the depressant effects of alcohol.

4. There is no indication that a spinal tap is needed.

Nursing Process: Planning

Client Need: Physiological Integrity

1 1 - 4 9

② **The nurse should orient the client. Immediately after clients awaken following electro-convulsive therapy (ECT), they are confused and disoriented. The nurse's orientation should be brief, distinct, and easy to comprehend.**

1. Just because a client is awake does not mean that the gag reflex has returned. Until the client's gag reflex returns, nothing should be eaten. The client should not be served until oriented, coordinated, and able to manage the diet.

3. Clients are too confused immediately after awakening from ECT to contemplate suicide.

4. A quiet environment is helpful but it would not be the first priority.

Nursing Process: Implementing

Client Need: Psychosocial Integrity

11-50

① **The nurse should tell the mother that the "little white spots" are called milia and that they will soon disappear. The white spots are due to retention of sebaceous material within the sebaceous gland. Milia are clinically insignificant and disappear during the neonatal period.**

2. Telling the client, "Most babies have them; there is no need to worry," does not answer the mother's question.

3. Milia are not cysts. Telling a client not to be concerned without answering the question will block further communication and disregards the client's concerns.

4. Telling a mother, "Some babies have more spots than your baby," conveys that the client should not complain since other babies are "worse off."

Nursing Process: Implementing
Client Need: Psychosocial Integrity

Practice Test 12

Miscellaneous Questions

1 2 - 1

When providing assistance at the site of an accident, the nurse should understand that the chief purpose of Good Samaritan laws is to:

1. discourage lay people from giving first aid to accident victims.
2. encourage health professionals to give first aid at the scene of an accident.
3. require licensed health practitioners to provide first aid to persons in medical emergencies.
4. make it compulsory for the injured person to accept first aid.

1 2 - 2

A nurse is to administer 50 mg of a 100-mg premeasured ampule of meperidine. The nurse administering this medication knows the unused portion should be:

1. placed in the refrigerator with the client's name and room number clearly visible.
2. disposed of in the presence of a second nurse witness and documented on the medication record.
3. returned to the pharmacy and credited to the client's account.
4. returned to a locked cabinet where all controlled medications are kept.

1 2 - 3

At the scene of an automobile accident, which of the following actions is most appropriate to take prior to the arrival of the emergency services?

1. Identify the client.
2. Apply firm pressure over cuts and abrasions to stop bleeding.
3. Immobilize the victim in the position found at the site of the accident.
4. Keep the victim warm and calm.

1 2 - 4

An 18-month-old is placed in a mist tent. Because the child continually tries to get out of the mist tent, soft restraints are applied. As a consequence of applying restraints, which of the following nursing actions is essential?

1. Tell the client's mother that bilateral arm and leg restraints are necessary for toddlers.

2. Inform the client's mother that the client will probably adjust better to the restraints if left alone for a while after they are applied.

3. Explain to the child's mother the need for restraints in order to help her accept the use of them on her child.

4. Observe the client after applying restraints to determine if he struggles to the point of negating the value of the therapy.

1 2 - 5

A mother of a 1-year-old and a 3-year-old is talking with the nurse about the eating habits of her children. When comparing the eating habits of typical children of these ages, which of the following differences are likely to be evident?

1. The food intake of a 3-year-old will be about 3 times greater that that of the 1-year-old.

2. A 1-year-old will have stronger preferences than a 3-year-old.

3. A 3-year-old will do more fingering of foods than a 1-year-old.

4. The appetite of a 3-year-old is likely to be more capricious than that of a 1-year-old.

1 2 - 6

You are assessing developmental achievements in an 18-month-old. You will expect to observe which of the following abilities in a normal 18-month-old child?

1. to stand briefly on one foot without support and to put together a simple jigsaw puzzle

2. to drink through a straw and to know own sex

3. to manage finger foods and to understand "No! No!"

4. to build a tower of 7 blocks and to open doors by turning knobs

1 2 - 7

The mother of a premature infant asks the nurse when her baby will be fed for the first time. To respond appropriately, the nurse must know that the feeding method used and the time of the first feeding is based chiefly on the premature infant's:

1. birth weight.
2. degree of hydration.
3. level of physiologic maturity.
4. total body surface.

1 2 - 8

Immediately after the death of a client, which of the following actions would be important for the nurse to perform first?

1. Pad all orifices of the body.
2. Place the body in a normal anatomical position.
3. Assemble the personal effects for the family.
4. Put the identification tags on the body.

1 2 - 9

Assessment is the first step in the nursing process and is best described as:

1. determining the effectiveness of therapy.
2. action oriented.
3. collection of the client's health data.
4. establishing goals.

1 2 - 1 0

The nurse is recording early morning care. An error is made while charting a narrative statement. The best way to correct this error is to:

1. cross out by making vertical and horizontal lines through the sentence.
2. tear out and rewrite the narrative.
3. erase completely and begin again.
4. draw a single horizontal line through the error and begin recording again.

12-11

An infant is born with superficial cracking of the skin, peeling, and lack of subcutaneous fat. These physical findings indicate:

1. appropriate for gestational age.
2. large for gestational age.
3. preterm.
4. postterm.

12-12

A 3-year-old presents to the Emergency Department with second-degree burns of the buttocks and lower extremities. The child's caretaker says, "I don't know how the child could have received these burns." The nurse has a responsibility to:

1. notify the Department of Social Services-Child Welfare.
2. notify the nursing supervisor.
3. notify the physician.
4. carefully document all findings.

12-13

The nurse is asked to be a witness when a client signs the consent form for a coronary artery angiography. Which of the following actions would be most important for the nurse to carry out?

1. Make certain that the client understands the procedure, including the risks.
2. Inform the client of the risks involved in the procedure.
3. Give the client an explanation of the medical aspects of the procedure.
4. Have the client sign the consent form immediately before the procedure.

12-14

Which of the following behaviors would the nurse expect an 8-week-old infant to exhibit during hospitalization?

1. assume a less-flexed position when prone
2. roll over from back to side
3. sit in a high chair with back straight
4. sit alone steadily

12-15

The nurse receives a call from a parent stating her child ingested an unknown amount of kerosene that had been stored in a carbonated drink can. The immediate first aid response will include:

1. giving ipecac to induce vomiting.
2. calling emergency 911.
3. contacting the poison control center.
4. observing the child's level of consciousness.

12-16

In planning the care for a 12-year-old, a nurse will consider which of the following behaviors for this age group?

1. rejects new routines
2. is eager to meet new people
3. is anxious when separated from parents
4. needs privacy

12-17

Which of the following behaviors would give the best indication that long-term adjustment is favorable in a toddler with a chronic disease?

1. eating habits improve
2. weight gain is appropriate for the toddler's age
3. interacts in a positive manner with peers
4. does not display signs and symptoms of the illness

12-18

You would like to suggest making changes in how assignments are determined. The best approach to creating the necessary climate for change is to:

1. meet with the charge nurse and arrive at an agreement.
2. post a notice requesting signatures of those in favor of the idea.
3. gain the support of one peer at a time.
4. present the relevant facts to those affected.

12-19

The nurse is assessing a newborn for the first time. Which finding should the nurse report to the physician immediately?

1. temperature of 97.8°F, respirations of 54 breaths per minute with periods of transient breathing, pulse rate of 142 beats per minute
2. passage of a large black stool
3. cyanosis of hands and feet
4. widening of the nares with inspiration and respiration of 76 breaths per minute

12-20

You are screening a client for lead poisoning. Due to developmental characteristics, which age group has the greatest need to be screened for lead poisoning?

1. toddlers
2. preschoolers
3. school-age children
4. adolescents

Practice Test 12

Answers, Rationales, and Explanations

1 2 - 1

② **Good Samaritan laws have been enacted in almost every state and territory to encourage health-care professionals to assist in emergency situations. These laws limit liability and offer legal immunity for people who help in an emergency, providing they give the best possible care under the conditions of the emergency.**

1. Good Samaritan laws were not enacted to discourage lay people but to encourage health professionals to give first aid at the scene of an accident.

3. Health professionals are not required by law to give assistance at an accident.

4. Good Samaritan laws were not enacted to require injured persons to accept first aid.

Nursing Process: Analyzing

Client Need: Safe, Effective Care Environment

1 2 - 2

② **The unused portion of a controlled medication should be disposed of in the presence of a second nurse witness and the amount wasted and the time documented on the medication record.**

1, 3, and 4. Placing the unused portion in the refrigerator, returning the unused portion to the pharmacy, or returning the medication to the medication box is inappropriate. Meperidine is a narcotic and is governed by federal law.

Nursing Process: Implementing

Client Need: Safe, Effective Care Environment

1 2 - 3

③ **It is important to immobilize victims of a car accident at the scene before the emergency medical services arrive. Due to potential spinal cord injury, the victim should be immobilized prior to any attempts to move or transport.**

1. Identifying the client is not the immediate concern.

2. Applying firm pressure over cuts and abrasions to stop bleeding could cause spinal cord injury if the client has not been immobilized.

4. Keeping the victim warm and calm should be done, but this would not be the first objective.

Nursing Process: Implementing

Client Need: Safe, Effective Care Environment

12-4

④ **The nurse should observe the child after restraints have been applied to determine if the client struggles to the point of negating the value of the therapy. A child in respiratory distress who is struggling to get out of restraints may compromise his or her condition by increasing oxygen demands.**

1. It is not necessary for a toddler to have 4-point restraints. Many times, a jacket restraint is sufficient. This will allow for self-consoling sucking of thumb or finger.
2. Children who require restraints will benefit from the presence of their parents.
3. All procedures should be explained. However, making sure that the restraints are not counterproductive is the most important consideration.

Nursing Process: Implementing

Client Need: Health Promotion and Maintenance

12-5

④ **The appetite of a 3-year-old is likely to be more capricious (unpredictable) than that of a 1-year-old.**

1. The 3-year-old is often a finicky eater with strong food preferences and decreased appetite.
2. The 1-year-old has a ferocious appetite and few food preferences.
3. The 1-year-old will do more fingering of foods than a 3-year-old.

Nursing Process: Analyzing

Client Need: Health Promotion and Maintenance

12-6

③ **The motor activity and cognitive ability to manage finger foods and to understand "No! No!" should be developed by 8 to 12 months. The other choices are tasks a 3-year-old should accomplish.**

1, 2, and 4. 3-year-olds should be able to stand briefly on one foot without support, put a simple jigsaw puzzle together, drink through a straw, know their own sex, build a tower of 7 blocks, and open doors by turning knobs.

Nursing Process: Analyzing

Client Need: Health Promotion and Maintenance

1 2 - 7

③ **The method used and the time of the first feeding for a premature infant is based on the infant's level of physiologic maturity. The sucking and swallowing reflexes of many preterm babies are insufficiently developed to enable sucking from either breast or bottle.**

1, 2, and 4. Determining when to administer the first feeding to a premature infant is not determined by the infant's birth weight, degree of hydration, or total body surface.

Nursing Process: Assessing
Client Need: Health Promotion and Maintenance

1 2 - 8

② **Immediately after death, the nurse should place the body of the deceased in a normal anatomical position. After death, the body undergoes many changes, including contraction of skeletal smooth muscle (rigor mortis). The care of the body should occur as soon as possible after death to prevent damage to tissues or disfigurement of body parts.**

1. It is not necessary to pad all body orifices. However, it may be necessary to place an absorbent pad under the buttocks of the deceased to collect any feces or urine that may be released when sphincter muscles relax.

3. All jewelry should be removed and personal effects gathered for the family; however, this is not the first priority.

4. Two identification tags (one tied to the big toe and one tied to the hand or wrist) should be placed on the deceased. However, this is not the first priority.

Nursing Process: Implementing
Client Need: Physiological Integrity

1 2 - 9

③ **Assessment involves the collection of data from sources such as the nursing history, health examination, review of records, consultation with staff members, and review of literature.**

1. Evaluating is the last phase of the nursing process and is concerned with the effectiveness of therapy.

2. The words "action oriented" describe the implementing phase of the nursing process.

4. The planning phase of the nursing process is concerned with the nurse's establishment of goals.

Nursing Process: Assessing
Client Need: Health Promotion and Maintenance

12-10

④ **Draw a single horizontal line through the error and begin recording again.**

1. It is not necessary to make both horizontal and vertical lines through a charting error.

2 and 3. Tearing out a charting error or erasing errors is not responsible nursing and it could bring the nurse's credibility into question. Also, the charting of other health-care providers may be on the same page. In a lawsuit, the client's attorneys could use a single improper correction to compromise a nurse's credibility. One improper correction could cast doubt on the entire chart.

Nursing Process: Evaluating
Client Need: Safe, Effective Care Environment

12-11

④ **Physical findings of post term infants include skin that is dry, cracked, thin, and peeling with very little subcutaneous fat; little vernix caseosa (except skin creases); a large amount of scalp hair; and yellow or green staining of skin, nails, and cord.**

1. The skin of a fullterm newborn should be the color consistent with genetic background, good turgor, without peeling and cracking. Subcutaneous fat should be present (appropriate for gestational age).

2. The skin of infants who are large for gestational age (LGA) has no cracking or peeling. There is, however, a greater amount of subcutaneous tissue and the infant's weight is above the 90 percentile on the weight and gestational age chart.

3. The skin of the preterm infant is reddened and translucent with blood vessels readily visible. There is also a lack of subcutaneous fat.

Nursing Process: Assessing
Client Need: Physiological Integrity

12-12

① **The nurse has the responsibility to notify the Department of Social Services-Child Welfare. It is mandatory in most states that the nurse report any suspected child abuse findings to child welfare.**

2. Notifying the nursing supervisor is proper protocol but is not essential.

3. Notifying the physician affords good communication and protocol but is not required.

4. Documentation is important for legal investigation in relation to abuse and the documentation should be specific and factual. This is second only to reporting suspected child abuse to child welfare.

Nursing Process: Planning
Client Need: Health Promotion and Maintenance

1 2 - 1 3

① **The nurse should make certain that the client understands the procedure, including the risks. Before witnessing a client's signature on the consent form, the nurse should confirm that the client is well informed, including understanding the risks of the procedure.**

2 and 3. It is the physician's responsibility to inform the client of the benefits and risks of surgery and anesthesia.

4. The consent form should not be signed immediately prior to the procedure. It should be signed in an unhurried atmosphere after having had the procedure and risks explained to the client's satisfaction.

Nursing Process: Implementing
Client Need: Safe, Effective Care Environment

1 2 - 1 4

① **The nurse would expect an 8-week-old infant to assume a less-flexed position when the infant is prone.**

2. Rolling over from back to side would occur at approximately 4 months of age.

3. Sitting in a high chair with the infant's back straight would occur at approximately 4 to 8 months of age.

4. Sitting alone steadily would occur at approximately 4 to 8 months of age.

Nursing Process: Implementing
Client Need: Physiological Integrity

1 2 - 1 5

③ **The parents should always call the poison control center to ask for advice on how to proceed when a poisonous substance has been ingested regardless if the amount of the substance is known or unknown.**

1. To induce vomiting would be contraindicated since kerosene (a petroleum-based substance) would burn as it comes up just as it did going down.

2. Emergency procedures outlined by the poison control center may be implemented while awaiting a 911 response.

4. Pharyngeal edema (obstruction of the airway that may lead to respiratory distress) will need to be assessed as well as the child's level of consciousness. However, calling the poison control center is the first priority.

Nursing Process: Evaluating
Client Need: Safe, Effective Care Environment

12-16

④ **Twelve-year-olds need privacy. They are entering puberty and may be self-conscious about secondary sex characteristics that are developing.**

1. Clients in early adolescence (11 to 14 years) are willing, if not eager, to try different things. They are not likely to reject new routines.

2. Clients in early adolescence (11 to 14 years) are generally shy, awkward, and feel more confident with same-sex friends.

3. Clients in early adolescence (11 to 14 years) are seeking emancipation from their parents and are not normally anxious when separated from them.

Nursing Process: Planning

Client Need: Health Promotion and Maintenance

12-17

② **The best indication that a toddler is adjusting favorably to a chronic disease would be body weight within normal range for the toddler's age.**

1. Improvement in the toddler's eating habits is a positive sign. However, sustained improved eating habits that lead to proper weight are the best indicators of a toddler's favorable adjustment to a chronic disease.

3. The toddler interacting in a positive manner with peers would indicate favorable short-term adjustment.

4. A toddler not displaying signs and symptoms of the disease would indicate a favorable short-term adjustment.

Nursing Process: Evaluating

Client Need: Health Promotion and Maintenance

12-18

④ **Change theory states that people affected by a change need to have all relevant information presented to them for a change to occur. A meeting of all people affected is a helpful way to discuss change. This way, all those affected will be present and able to discuss issues openly.**

1. The charge nurse is only one person who could be affected by change. All the people who could be affected should be informed.

2. Posting a notice requesting signatures is not in keeping with proper protocol and may be interpreted as a threat.

3. When making changes, it's best for all people involved to hear and discuss the issues in the same meeting. This leaves little room for misunderstanding and coercion.

Nursing Process: Planning

Client Need: Psychosocial Integrity

12-19

④ **Widening of the nares with 76 breaths per minute indicates respiratory distress and should be reported to the physician immediately.**

1. A temperature of 97.8°F, respirations of 54 breaths per minute with periods of transient breathing, and a pulse rate of 142 beats per minute indicates that vital signs are within normal limits.

2. Passage of 1 large black stool is normal meconium in the newborn infant.

3. Cyanosis of hands and feet are normal findings in a newborn infant. Acrocyanosis means a dark blue color and is normal the first hour of life.

Nursing Process: Analyzing

Client Need: Physiological Integrity

12-20

① **Toddlers have the greatest need to be screened for lead poisoning because of the possibility of brain damage. Lead poisoning is usually the result of pica (a perversion of appetite with ingestion of material not fit for food, such as clay, ice, starch, and plaster). Toddlers have a tendency to put inappropriate substances into their mouths.**

2, 3, and 4. Preschoolers, school-age children, and adolescents are not as likely to put inappropriate substances into their mouths as toddlers.

Nursing Process: Analyzing

Client Need: Health Promotion and Maintenance